Choose

Happiness

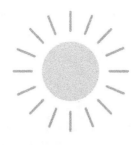

Choose Happiness

Rachel Cole

Front cover design by Sarah Cole.

www.choose-happiness.net

ISBN 978-0-578-82169-6

BOOK DESIGN BY RAESE DESIGN
Text set in Adobe Caslon

Dedicated to you, the reader.
May you always find a way to
choose happiness.

Contents

Author's Note

Welcome to *Choose Happiness*! Why a book devoted to this concept? Well, there's a lot of negativity out in the world and it's very easy to get caught up in it. Have you ever noticed that it's easier to focus on all of the bad stuff going on and the good stuff gets harder and harder to find? It's easy to be happy when things are going well for us, but for those times when we're stuck in difficult situations, I wondered if it was possible to make the choice to be happy and find joy in spite of our current less-than-ideal circumstances. I learned a long time ago that we get no "points" in life for suffering, and that it's one hundred percent up to us how happy or unhappy we choose to be on a daily basis. I also learned that no one and no one thing can make us happy or unhappy, it's truly up to us to make the choice every single day.

This concept was crystallized for me during a routine trip to the post office. I'm sort of friends with most of the people who work there (since I go there a lot) and Bill was one of the workers there who always had a smile on his face and was always ready with a joke or some good-natured teasing about the mountains of packages I was usually sending. On this occasion I was waiting in line with a bunch of other people, and a customer up at the counter started screaming angrily at Bill. She was clearly furious about something that had gone wrong, and she spent the next several minutes raging directly in Bill's face. Bill, meanwhile, was calmly nodding sympathetically, giving her suggestions about what she could do, and apologizing repeatedly for whatever had happened. She finally finished her rant and stormed out, and when I got up to the counter I said to Bill, "Wow, that was really something, how did you manage to keep it together so well?" And he replied, "Happiness is a choice. I'm not going to let a total stranger ruin my day."

Wow. He was so right. Why should any of us let anyone else steal our joy away for any reason? Happiness IS indeed a choice, and one that we can make at any moment during our lives depending on how we choose to look at things.

Happiness is also not something to be found sometime in the future. So often we get stuck in the mindset of "When I fall in love," or "When I finally have the perfect house," or "When I land my dream job," THEN I'll be happy. But we can't spend our lives chasing it, nor have our happiness depend on all of those external contrivances. Now is all we have, and any true and lasting happiness must come from within ourselves.

Choosing happiness is not an easy thing to do, and it does not mean putting our proverbial heads in the proverbial sand and ignoring the difficult things around us. We are all faced with a lot of challenges on our life's journeys and choosing happiness doesn't mean simply ignoring the things we don't like or the things that we have to do that may not bring us joy. Hopefully this book can be a tool to provide some ideas and strategies to help us navigate those tough times and remind us that no matter what is going on around us, we have control over how we choose to deal with it.

NOTE: This book is not necessarily meant to be read in order. Of course you are welcome to do that, but my hope is that when you need some encouragement or a reminder to choose happiness, you will be able to open up this book and find the exact right chapter or quote that you need at the exact right time. That's the intention, and although I hope you don't need it often, this will be right here for you when you do.

I, not events, have the power to make me happy or unhappy today. I can choose which it shall be. Yesterday is dead, tomorrow hasn't arrived yet. I have just one day, today, and I'm going to be happy in it.

—GROUCHO MARX

Happy Shoes

Here's a simple thing you can do to instantly perk up your day and tangibly remind yourself that you have power over your situation.

I call it: Happy Shoes.

Have something that makes you happy when you wear it—shoes, a shirt, a pair of funny socks—and keep it at the ready for when your spirit needs lifting, and, more importantly, to actively exert your own power over your current situation.

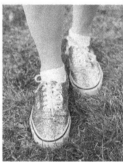

For example, I have happy shoes. I have one pair for the spring and summer that look like this (top):

And one pair for the fall and winter that look like this (bottom):

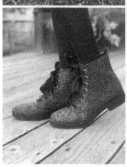

These glittery shoes always pick me up, and even just seeing them in my closet can bring me out of a bad mood. Wearing them puts a spring in my step—sometimes even literally—and I find that I'm able to see all of the good around me easily when I have my happy shoes on.

This concept comes from when I was in college and I met a girl, Susie, who was wearing a big colorful skirt with ruffles and flowers all over it. I said to her, "Wow, I love your skirt!" and she responded with, "Thanks! This is my happy skirt." And I was like, "What do you mean?" and she said, "When I'm really stressed our or feeling down I put on this skirt and it instantly cheers me up." I remember thinking to myself, "That's BRILLIANT!"

This concept has stuck with me for all of these years, and on the one hand, it's something very simple that works magnificently: We wear something that evokes happiness within ourselves to help us to be happy. But I have found that it's also something very empowering and profound. When you put on what you have deemed your "Happy Something" you are making the conscious choice to rise above your circumstances and how you are feeling about it. You remind yourself that while you may not have control over what is going on, you DO have control over how you are going to handle it. The great thing about this is that it's a tangible thing you can do to keep yourself from getting mired down in the despair or hopelessness that you may be feeling, plus it allows you to move along in your day with a spark of happiness to keep you where you want to be mentally and emotionally.

Try it! Find yourself something that you can assign the "Happy ____" moniker to and make the choice to put it on when you're feeling less happy than you'd like to be. And if someone compliments you on it, feel free to pass along the concept so they can take part in it as well. You never know how that might impact someone's life the way my encounter with Susie changed mine.

Thank you, Susie, wherever you are, for teaching me a fun and meaningful way to choose happiness in my life!

Always Have Something to Look Forward To

If there is one thing I could say that could pretty much guarantee happiness, it would be this:

Always have something to look forward to.

Having something you are looking forward to doing or experiencing can often make the difference between a good day and a bad day. It can be something small, like meeting friends for coffee or going for a haircut; it can be big, like a trip overseas or a new job; or it can be anything in-between.

When you are in the state of anticipating something that you are going to enjoy, it instantly makes you hopeful and happy. Just thinking about and planning whatever it is can fill us with endorphins and help to mentally take ourselves out of a difficult situation if we're in one.

The funny thing is, sometimes the "looking forward to" part ends up being even better than the actual thing you do! I've heard that about vacations, parties, concerts, and special events. But even if the thing you were looking forward to is a letdown, at least you had all of the time beforehand to be happy while you were expecting, planning, and hoping for something wonderful.

Studies on happiness have shown that the more we have to look forward to, the more positive our lives become overall. Think about children on Christmas Eve, who are bursting with joyous anticipation for the next morning. Can you imagine feeling that way every day, or at least on as many days as possible? ALWAYS have something to look forward to, even if it's just a hot bath after a long day of work or an ice cream cone after the drudgery of cleaning out the garage. Make that choice, and the happiness you feel will be what helps you keep going forward with optimism, regardless of how the actual thing you looked forward to turns out.

> *Looking forward to things is half the pleasure of them.*
> *You mayn't get the things themselves;*
> *but nothing can prevent you from having the fun*
> *of looking forward to them.*
> —L. M. Montgomery

What are you looking forward to? Whatever it is, I hope you choose to enjoy every moment leading up to it, as well as the next one that happily comes along.

Celebrate Everything!

I was just watching Ina Garten on a CBS *Sunday Morning* segment, and she signed off by saying, "Celebrate everything!"

This really resonated with me, because I have long been a proponent of celebrating anything and everything. I have always loved throwing parties, which explains both why my oft-desired gift as a young child was always a tea set, the more cups and saucers the better!

There's a reason why most cultures have celebratory rituals that include gatherings of people for significant life transitions like wedding and funeral rites. Many faith practices have requirements for praying together in a community because the power of collective worship elevates the soul and helps participants to feel connected on a spiritual level.

Any kind of coming together for a single purpose can be powerful and energizing, for people of all ages. I was a professional events planner for many years, and then channeled my party planning passion into events for my kids as well as family and friends. In our house we always celebrate special occasions but have also been known to throw impromptu gatherings just for fun.

I personally feel that one of my life callings is to actively bring people together to celebrate things, whether for special commemorative purposes, or for no reason other than we're glad and grateful to be alive.

Be the celebrators, celebrate! Already there is too much—
the flowers have bloomed, the birds are singing, the sun is
there in the sky—celebrate it! You are breathing and you
are alive and you have consciousness, celebrate it!
—Osho, *Creativity: Unleashing the Forces Within*

I encourage you to connect with other people and celebrate the fact that no matter what may be going on in the world around us, there is always something to be grateful for. Find that and celebrate it. Make the choice to celebrate everything!

Joie de Vivre

A few years ago, my family and I traveled to Europe, and the highlight of the trip was spending a day in a beautiful town outside of Paris called Nemours. We met up with the most gracious family we have ever known (shout out to John Hochart and family!) and after a wonderful day of visiting sites and enjoying time together, we set off on an evening walking tour of the neighborhood. A few blocks in we walked past a street-level garage with the door open. Inside was a large table, surrounded by about ten people, all of whom were eating, laughing, and talking merrily. They were noisy, they were happy, and they were having a fabulous time. More than two hours later, as we came back that way and approached the open door, we heard snatches of song and uproarious laughter. Sure enough, as we went by, the people were still at their table, eating and drinking, and still having a splendidly glorious time. We waved at them and they waved back, and some raised their glasses and shouted something gleeful at us. We couldn't help smiling and marveling at their continued revelry.

While I only got a quick look into the garage, I could see that that there was no Pinterest-inspired centerpiece in the middle of the table, nor were there expensive-looking plates and perfectly matching glasses. No one was dressed up, it wasn't a special occasion, it was simply Tuesday evening dinner. What also struck me was that no one was on their phone, no one was posing for a photo, and no one seemed to be worrying about what was to come tomorrow. Everyone was just completely in the moment, enjoying good food and drink, and basking in each other's company. It almost felt miraculous, seeing the people in this eleventh-century town, who were able to capture what is truly important, and who were choosing to savor the joy that life can bring on a daily basis.

That fleeting experience has stayed with me for all of these years, and I hearken back to it often, especially when I am feeling concern about what my house looks like if someone stops by unannounced or when I set the table for a dinner party and find that my cloth napkins are fraying at the edges. I remind myself of those cheerful people, living life to the fullest, and not caring about what was on the table more than who was around it. They were making the choice to be happy in the presence of their loved ones and making the absolute most and best of the time they had together. They had true joie de vivre, which is defined as "exuberant enjoyment of life."

Let's choose THAT, as often as we can, shall we?

The Time Is Going to Pass Anyway

I saw a segment on TV recently that changed my life. A journalist was interviewing a man in his forties and he was talking about how when he had just finished college his dream was to go to medical school and become a doctor. He wasn't able to pursue that dream at the time, but when he turned forty he realized that now he had both the means and the time to finally make this dream come true.

When he told people about his plans to go to medical school at age forty, one person said to him, "But that's seven years of your life! It's going to take so much time!"

The man replied, "Well, those seven years are going to pass anyway, I might as well spend it doing what I've always wanted to do."

The time is going to pass anyway.

What an amazing concept! How often do we talk ourselves out of doing something that we have always wanted to do because we think it will take a long time?

(Which, by the way, the worthwhile things usually do.)

We have to remind ourselves that while yes, it will probably take a long time and even be difficult at times, however long it takes, the time will pass anyway. When we think about that, we can also ask ourselves, if we're not pursuing our lifelong dream, how else would we be spending that time? Binge-watching another television show? Endlessly scrolling on social media watching what other people are doing? Sitting at home doing the same thing day after day, wishing desperately that we were doing something more fulfilling?

I know a lot of people who use time as a reason, or more accurately, as an excuse, for not achieving their goals. But here's the thing about time:

It's fixed. We all get the same number of minutes and seconds and hours in a day. We don't have any control over how quickly time passes or how it passes at all. What we DO have control over is how we spend it.

It has been said that if you want to see what truly matters to a person, look at how they spend their money and how they spend their time. People can say that something means a lot to them, but if they aren't consciously spending time on it then how important is it to them really? We make time for the things that matter, and often mindlessly fill our time with things that don't, but that is a choice too. We're choosing to actively NOT spend our time doing what we really want, and then use "I don't have time" as a justification for our fear or trepidation.

So the next time you think you don't have time to pursue something that will make you happy, or you think that taking a lot of time to do something that will ultimately bring you joy will take too long, remember the words of that wise medical student:

The time is going to pass anyway. You might as well spend it doing what you've always wanted to do.

Move Your Body

... and I would add to that, ANY WAY YOU WANT TO.

A guaranteed way to keep your mind and spirit happy is to keep your body happy, which translates to keeping it healthy and strong. There are thousands of studies that show how vitally important exercise is for our physical health, and that it also plays a key role in keeping our mental state bright and balanced overall. According to science, as well as from personal experience, it seems that nothing beats regular exercise as a practice to keep us on the road to happiness within ourselves and with the world around us.

Unfortunately, the capital E "Exercise" can sometimes be daunting, and the way that it is presented to us can sometimes look scary and even impossible. The truth is, all we have to do is get our heart rate up and make our muscles strong, and there are an infinite number of ways to get both of those things accomplished. We do not have to join a gym and do so many reps on a machine or go a certain distance on a treadmill if these things do not personally resonate with us and keep us joyful.

So I say, take the pressure off! Take the word "Exercise" out of your vocabulary and get your mind off of what has been fed to us as to what moving our bodies has to look like to "count." Remove the external mandate of the outside world telling us this is something that we "Have to Do," and change it to something that we "Choose to Do," because it's fun and because we like the way we feel when we're doing it.

I personally can't do high-impact things like running or jumpy aerobics because of a back injury and a chronically inflamed Achilles tendon. What I CAN do, and that I enjoy doing, are swimming, walking, hiking, dancing, and doing my old Dancerobics tapes on low impact. (No judgment here please!) I also work out with light weights and do a circuit of sit-ups, push-ups, lunges and other calisthenics, along with stretching (which I always seem to need to do more of). None of these activities require a gym membership (except the swimming) and I look forward to them every day, especially the days when I just crank up the music and have a rockin' dance party for one in my bedroom with the door closed. Getting sweaty and having that wonderful release of endorphins in our brains and bodies can go a very long way when we're feeling down or need to boost our spirits.

For you, moving your body could be getting your heart rate up on an elliptical machine, taking a Pilates class, or doing goat or puppy yoga. It might be meeting your friends every week for a jog or a pickup game of basketball or soccer. Maybe it's riding horses or doing water aerobics, or ice-skating. Whatever it is, pick something that you love doing so you'll make sure to keep doing it and having it bring you joy.

Moving our bodies doesn't have to be a big deal, it can just be something fun that we choose to do to keep ourselves healthy and happy.

Choose to be happy.

That is the only way to find happiness.

—DEBASISH MRIDHA

Change Your Password

I read about this idea a few years ago and I love it because it's one of those little things than can actually make a seismic shift in our mindset each day.

I'm a big believer in posting positive messages on the bathroom mirror and giving ourselves encouragement on a daily basis. One of the best ways to do this is to change the password on your computer to something very specific that relates to a goal you want to accomplish. How many times do we log onto our computers in one day? It can be up to twenty times or more for some of us. Wouldn't it be incredible to have something uplifting and inspiring greeting us that many times while masquerading as a menial task?

There is a cognitive link between writing something down and our brains believing it. This is why the action of actually writing out our goals, either with a pen and paper or on a typewriter or computer, can be so powerful. The trick is, it works best if you write out the goal *as if it has already happened.*

In the original article I read, a man was struggling with forgiving his ex-wife. So he decided to change his computer password to "I forgive Jo." He typed it multiple times a day, and after about a week of this he found his attitude shifting toward forgiveness and peace about his divorce rather than the rage and anger that was his first instinct. Actually typing out the words, and saying them to himself as he did so, made a huge change in his life and his daily well-being. He hadn't forgiven his wife when he started, but by telling himself that he had, he began to believe it, which manifested itself in it actually happening.

Pretty cool, huh?

So how can we do this for ourselves for the things we want to accomplish in our own lives? Let's say that one of your dreams is to be a writer. Change your password to "I am a writer." Not "I want to be a writer" or "I wish I was a writer," but "I AM A WRITER." Try that for a week or two and see what happens. If you want to be a singer, a chef, an accountant, a scientist, or whatever other dream occupation you have, try putting in that job title and see how it makes you feel.

Maybe one of your goals is something less tangible than that. Maybe you're struggling with long-held beliefs about yourself that you want to shed. Try changing your password to "I AM ENOUGH," or "I AM BEAUTIFUL," or "I AM WORTHY," or "I AM LOVED."

If one of your goals is to choose happiness on a daily basis, then your password can simply be "I AM HAPPY." Type that in multiple times a day and I can promise you, your life will change for the better. This small, conscious act can honestly make all the difference in you taking control of your happiness journey.

Find Your Happy Place

It is so important to have a "Happy Place" that you can visit both physically and, when necessary, in your mind.

My happy place is the ocean. Whenever I'm able to be by the ocean it fills me up with happiness and peace. There's something about watching the waves crash upon the sand repeatedly that brings me a beautiful sense of tranquility and inspiration. Maybe it's because I can see them and remember that these same waves were hitting the sand for millions of years before I existed, and the tides will continue to ebb and flow for millions of years after my time on Earth has ended, and that reminder gives me a beautiful perspective of my place in the world and can also spur me on to accomplish my goals while I'm still here.

Even just hearing the waves and breathing the salt-scented air brings me joy, which is why I try to get to the ocean as often as I can. When I can't get there often in person, I can return there in my mind, picturing the sparkling water and the foamy surf and feeling the ocean breeze ruffling my hair and cooling my face. It's a great place to go to while meditating or when I'm trying to fall asleep as well.

The mountains are a happy place for a lot of people. I think there's a similar sense of these colossal, naturally made masses, that have been here for eons and will continue to stand magnificently for eons more, that allow people to relax and feel connected to nature while they are hiking or skiing or just spending time away from an industrialized place. Even just seeing pictures of mountains can help people get out of the daily grind and take our minds on a beautiful trip to someplace untouched by the rigors or ennui of our routine.

Any place can be a happy place. Some people (me included) love the quiet and orderliness of a library. Some people (me included) love browsing through bookstores, especially the ones that have overflowing shelves and floor stacks of used books. One person's happy place might be performing on a stage to an appreciative audience, one might be up in a drafty attic garret writing poetry. Do you love holding and being around infants? A lot of hospitals have a Cuddle Program where you can volunteer to hold babies in the NICU. (I'll tell you, there's nothing like holding a sleeping baby in your arms to remind you that everything's going to be all right.)

Some people's happy place is the gym, where they can sweat their troubles away. For some it might be a skating rink, dance studio, a photography darkroom, sitting at a pottery wheel, or a standing at painting easel. For some it might be up in a tree, sitting on a favorite rock, or digging in a garden. Happy places don't have to be solitary—some people's happy places could be a tennis court, a football field, or in the stands of a crowded stadium cheering on their favorite sports team.

Feel free to think outside the box on this. Ask yourself, where is a place that I feel filled up and happy every time I go there? What is it about that place that brings me joy? Try to re-create it in your mind as clearly as possible, and when you're able to be there physically, try to bring back something to remind you of how you feel while you're there. If it's the beach, collect some sand in a jar or some seashells and keep them on your desk or nightstand to remind you of your happy place. If it's a lake or mountains, select a rock from the area and keep it nearby, in a pocket or a purse as a tangible reminder of the place where you feel happiest. Take photos of your happy place, print them out, and place them where you can see them often.

Wherever it is, have a happy place to return to in your mind when you need to, and I hope you get to go there as often as possible in person too.

Surround Yourself with Things You Love

A wonderful way to consciously choose happiness is to surround yourself with things you love. When you walk around your living space, the things that you see should bring you joy, regardless if they are what is "on trend" in the design world, if they match each other, or if they are what someone else says is "supposed" to be there.

Some years ago I knew a wealthy family who had recently moved into a neighboring town and the mom was having a hard time decorating the new house. At some point she hired an interior designer and spent weeks poring over things like custom cut tiles and hand-crafted kitchen drawer pulls. One day I got to see her new bedroom furniture. It was a set of enormous pieces in a very dark wood, some of which had custom designed fabric on it. (I have no idea what it cost but it looked really expensive.) I complimented it sincerely, because even though it wasn't my taste it was beautiful and exquisitely made. At one point I asked her, "Do you love it?"

She hesitated a moment, and then replied, "Ummm, well, not really."

"What?!" I asked, incredulously.

"Well, . . ." she began, "it's kind of big, and it's kind of dark … and it's not really my style."

"Oh," I said. "Sooo, why did you get it?"

She sighed and answered, "The decorator talked me into it. She said this is really trendy right now."

Maybe it was, but when she said that, two things came to mind. (1) If something is trendy at a certain point in time then that inherently means that one day soon it will no longer be trendy and something else will be en vogue. With clothes and accessories that's one thing, but with such a long-lasting purchase like furniture, should the trendiness of it be a major deciding factor? (2) The decorator wasn't going to be living in this house. In fact, she probably was never going to set foot into that house again, so why on earth would my friend make a decision that was going to last for decades based on what that person liked? Why would anyone?

I have an "art wall" in my house that is covered with my kids' artwork from their school assignments and projects from their younger school days. It makes me happy every time I see it, and it's a point of interest, like the concept of an accent wall in a room. I've had people come over and spend time looking at all of the art, smiling to themselves and occasionally asking me about some of the drawings or designs.

I have also had people come over, take one look at the wall, and say to me things like, "What the heck is THIS?" and "Why would you have this up in your house, your kids are older now." And, "When are you going to take this down, this is ridiculous."

First of all, I will never understand why unkind people will forever be convinced that their unsolicited and overwhelmingly negative opinions matter and need to be spoken aloud to whoever is within earshot. Secondly, I don't understand why someone who is visiting me for a few minutes or hours on one day feels the need to comment on how I choose to decorate my surroundings. Thirdly (and perhaps most importantly), I need to consider the source in these matters and definitely think twice before inviting these inconsiderate people back into my home.

The point is, regardless of what anyone else thinks or feels the need to say about your home space, decorate it the way that YOU like, with things that lift you up and bring you joy. You spend a lot of time in your personal space, so make sure that whatever is in it makes you happy.

The "I Am Happy" Exercise

My #1 favorite comedian of all time, Jake Johannsen, tells a great story about how his three-year-old daughter was sitting in her high-chair one morning, when all of a sudden she announces loudly, "I AM HAPPY." Jake looks at her, takes it in for moment, and answers her, "I AM HAPPY TOO." Then he and his wife and their little girl all smile at each other, and he shares that it was as if time stood still for the next few seconds. It was a transformative experience in his life, which he shares with his audience, and he even had t-shirts made up with the phrase "I am happy," on it (one of which I am a proud owner).

Why did this simple statement from a toddler make such an impact on him? Because he realized how most young children are just naturally happy. They wake up, excited to have a brand-new day in front of them where they get to play and explore and learn and absolutely enjoy themselves. Everything is bright and new and theirs for the taking, and most young kids carry an optimism around with them that sadly gets taken away from them bit by bit as they get older and encounter stressful and difficult people and experiences.

But it wasn't only was the fact that his daughter was feeling unabashedly filled with joy. The more striking thing was that she stated it so clearly and succinctly to the world around her. It was like by saying it out loud, she was declaring it to be a beautifully factual statement.

Try it—try saying those words out loud right now:

"I am happy."

Now say it again:

"I am happy."

Say it one more time, just a little bit louder than the last time:

"I am happy."

How do you feel? A little bit happier maybe?

I believe that affirming something out loud that we want to be true can go a very long way in manifesting it for ourselves. What we say can really chart the course of our lives and our individual days and moments.

Imagine that you wake up and it's raining outside. If the first thing you say to yourself when you look out the window is "Oh no, it's raining! Now I'm going to get wet at the bus stop and I can't wear the shoes I was planning to wear and I have to find my umbrella and ugh, what a terrible day," I can tell you unequivocally that just by the simple act of you stating all of that you are setting yourself up for indeed an awful day to be had.

Let me make something clear here—the rain did not ruin your day, YOU did.

Now imagine that you wake up and it's raining outside. The first thing you say to yourself when you look out the window is "Oh cool, it's raining! Now my plants will get watered, the grass will be so green, and now I can wear rain boots to work and be so much more comfortable. What a great day!"

Seems simplistic, and maybe it is, but it's also super powerful.

We all set our intention for our day ahead without even realizing it. Can you imagine the kind of day you would have if you started every morning saying out loud, "I am happy."? Not only would you be proclaiming that objective for yourself right away, but chances are, even if little things went wrong throughout your morning—like the coffee maker wasn't working or you were out of toothpaste or the shirt you had planned on wearing was dirty—they might not affect you as negatively because you already told yourself you were happy. Little irritations might not bother you because your mindset was already in the mode of being positive and focused on joy. So if the coffee maker breaks it becomes "Yay, I get to treat myself to a coffee at the coffee shop!" If you run out of toothpaste your reaction becomes, "I've always heard of people using baking soda to brush their teeth, now's the perfect time for me to try that!" If the shirt you had planned on wearing is in the laundry bin then you can reach way back into the recesses of your closet and have a moment of "Oh yeah, I loved this top and used to wear it all the time but forgot about it. Cool!"

Here's a challenge for you: When you first wake up in the morning, say out loud to yourself, "I am happy." Have it be the very first thing you say. Try this for thirty days straight and see what happens. It might change your life; it might do nothing. But just try it and see. It certainly couldn't hurt, could it?

Don't Give Up So Easily

Yesterday morning I learned a great lesson in not giving up, and also in not beating myself up along the way.

In my continued quest to try cooking and baking things I've never made before, I decided to try making Swedish pancakes. I mixed up the batter, heated up the griddle, and proceeded to *kör på*! (go for it!)

First one: Into the garbage.

Second one: Into the garbage.

Third one: Was almost right, but ended up in the garbage.

Fourth one: Half into the garbage, the other half into my mouth, just to see what I was dealing with here.

Fifth one: Was just about right, and I ate it triumphantly with butter and syrup.

The rest of them turned out beautifully, and I saved them for my family for when they got up and made their way downstairs for breakfast. They were a big hit, and everyone asked if I would please make them again and soon.

Optimistically I said, "Of course!" but inside I was thinking to myself, "Maybe for a special occasion..."

Swedish pancakes are super light and thin, akin to crepes, but even more delicate. When you put the batter into the pan you have to swirl it around so that it reaches the edges and can cook evenly. My first four failures had many issues including too much butter in the pan, too much batter, too high of a heat, the wrong sized spatula, the list goes on. But I kept trying and eventually I figured out all of the elements for success in this endeavor. Like crepes, you have to make them one at a time, so it was quite an undertaking, but it was fun and I felt great at being able to master something new.

About the time that I was pouring out batter number twelve or so, I realized something. At no point during this process did I put myself down or feel badly about myself for not getting it right on the first try. I knew that with cooking, and especially with experimenting with a new recipe, there are many variables to consider when it comes to doing it correctly. I wasn't upset at all when I was tossing away those first few attempts; I used them to try to figure out how I could do it more effectively the next time.

Which totally worked! I know that these are only pancakes, but they can serve as a great metaphor for accomplishing things that we want to do in our lives. How many times have we given up because we couldn't get something on the first try? How many times have we tried something once or twice, didn't get the results we wanted, and abandoned the task altogether, along with all hope of ever achieving success?

It would have been really easy to just toss the batter and mix up my tried-and-true regular pancake recipe. But I had a whole bowlful of it, I had some time alone in the kitchen, and honestly it never occurred to me to give up. Not only would it have been wasteful, but I really thought that if I tried enough times and made adjustments along the way that I'd be able to do this successfully.

Patience, perseverance, and hard work are what make things happen in our lives. There are no shortcuts. As much as we might not want to have to try something hundreds of times before we get it right, that's often how it goes, and the final mastery of something is so much more rewarding after we've put in so much time and effort, isn't it?

While making Swedish pancakes is in no way on par with Edison creating the incandescent light bulb or the Wright brothers figuring out manned flight, the concept of trying new things, and then encouraging ourselves to keep going instead of putting ourselves down until we ultimately give up, is the same.

> *I have not failed,*
> *I've just found 10,000 ways that don't work.*
> —Thomas Edison

Most of the time when we fail at something it's due to mindset, not ability. Most of the time it's because we don't have the patience or the persistence to keep working at a task until we can finally get it right. Most of the time we spend so much time doubting ourselves or demeaning our lack of skills that we don't even notice the incremental progress we might have made. And most of the time we let the "I can't" take over the "I'll try" mentality that pervades so much of our daily attitude and psyche.

So if there is something you have always wanted to try doing, I encourage you to DO IT! Give yourself the time, the patience, and the strength to keep going if you don't get it right on the first few tries. I can guarantee that even if your first hundred proverbial pancakes go into the trash, you will keep learning and keep achieving, and your life will be richer and more satisfying as a result of your continued determination and belief in yourself.

There will always be a reason to give up. But there is also always a reason to keep trying. Which will you choose?

Be happy for this moment.

This moment is your life.

—OMAR KHAYYAM

How to Keep Your Sanity When You're in a Really Difficult Situation

If you find yourself in a situation that is hard to deal with, hopefully you can physically remove yourself from it. There are times when that is impossible, however, and in those times, here is something to try:

Take things one minute at a time.

If that seems impossible, take them one second at a time.

I have done this, and it can make all the difference between getting through something horrific … or not.

A few years ago, I had an absolutely terrible day. The details of it aren't important, but by the time I got to dinnertime, I felt like I was going to have a complete emotional breakdown.

Normally I would have removed myself from the situation, but for a variety of reasons that wasn't possible. To make things worse, I was in a very public place, so the things that probably would have made me feel better (screaming, crying, throwing things) were not possible. At the moment when I felt like I couldn't take it anymore, I came up with something that saved me from tipping over into hysterical despair.

I took things one minute at a time. Actually, for the first few minutes, I took things one second at a time. I became hyper-focused on what I was doing and didn't think about anything else. I remember I was eating a salad, and as all of the loud commotion of hundreds of people was going on around me, I said quietly to myself, "Right now I'm cutting this cucumber. Now the cucumber is cut. Now I'm going to bring it to my mouth. Now I'm chewing the cucumber. Now I'm swallowing the cucumber. Now I'm going to spear that tomato..."

It may sound crazy, but honestly, making the choice to concentrate completely on what I was doing in a slow and meditative manner calmed my nerves and mentally removed me from the untenable situation that I was unable to remove myself from physically. I felt my pulse and my blood pressure slow down, and after about five minutes or so of doing this, I was able to manage looking up from my plate and rejoining the world outside of my mind.

The same tactic can be used when facing a hard day ahead. I can remember waking up to a day that I knew was going to be extremely demanding emotionally. So I focused on whatever I was doing at the moment, quietly and deliberately. "Right now I'm squeezing the shampoo into my hand to wash my hair..." "Right now I'm putting on my right shoe, pulling the laces tightly and making a bow..." "Right now I'm getting into the car and putting on my seat belt..." and so on and so on. Keeping my brain and body fixated on only what I was doing, in every moment as the day went along, helped me to get done what needed to be done, and kept me on an even keel mentally.

While we may not have a choice to experience the times that try our patience and our very sanity, we can choose how we deal with them. We can choose to curl into a ball on the floor, we can choose to make a life-altering scene in a public place, or we can choose to do what we need to do to seize our own power over the situation and keep propelling ourselves forward in a healthy way. Sometimes that looks like taking one tiny step, followed by another nearly infinitesimal step, followed by another one, all the while keeping control over those steps until we get to where we need and want to be.

So when things seem impossible, take them a minute or a second at a time. The time will tick by and you will come out as a survivor on the other side.

Something That Can Keep You Happy for a Month

I recently saw Rainn Wilson from Soul Pancake (www.soul pancake.com) interview Dr. Laurie Santos. She's a professor at Yale who teaches the most popular course Yale has ever offered, called "Psychology and the Good Life,"* informally known as "Happiness 101." There are two specific tips that I wanted to share with you from that interview about how to bring more happiness into your life.

The first is called "The Three Blessings." Dr. Santos advises that each of us take time each day to come up with three things that make us happy or three things that we're grateful for. She stressed the importance of writing them down every time (either on paper or using our phones), both to make it something tangible and engaging our minds with our bodies, and also to have the things actually there for us to see in case we forget some of them. She suggested setting a phone alarm at the same time every day to make sure we do this or harnessing the exercise with a daily habit so it also becomes something that we do regularly. She does hers while brushing her teeth—it's two minutes of "free" time that she can use to focus on her three blessings of the day.

*As of this book's first printing, this course was being offered for free online through Yale under the name "The Science of Well-Being." https://www .coursera.org/learn/the-science-of-well-being.

The second also has an element of three to it—a hat trick contained in one thing. A lot of her teaching focuses on the importance of social interaction, especially since so much of our communication with friends and loved ones these days takes place over texts instead of meeting up face-to-face or even talking to each other on the phone. She cited data that says that loneliness and isolation can be as dangerous to our health as smoking fifteen cigarettes a day. So, if we're seeking happiness, we need to make sure to consciously create opportunities for sociability to happen.

When we're feeling down and need a lift to our spirits, we can call or meet up with someone we feel comfortable with. Having this interaction is #1, and just the act of connecting with someone in person or over the phone should make us feel happier overall. If that person isn't doing well, and we can do our part to serve them and help to lift them up, that can provide a huge boost to our own mood, which is #2. Studies have shown that contrary to popular belief, expending our efforts on others instead of demanding "me" time actually makes us exponentially happier than when we just focus on ourselves. The concept of being "otherish" (the opposite of "selfish") and looking outside of ourselves to provide for the needs of others gives us joy and satisfaction on a primal and anthropological level.

The third part of this, which really blew me away, is that when you express gratitude to this person—telling them how much you appreciate them and how glad you are to have them in your life—that simple act can lift your spirits and keep you happy for a month. A whole month! Is there anything else you can think of that can give you guaranteed happiness for a month?

Everyone is different, and not everyone will react to these practices the same way. But they are a great jumping-off point for those of us who might have trouble choosing happiness, especially when things aren't particularly going well for us in our lives, or when we find ourselves caught up in a monotonous daily or weekly routine.

So Happiness 101? Make and keep a list of what you're grateful for and happy about, and cultivate and maintain social interactions with people who are "nutritious" to you, whether it's them lifting you up, or you getting the benefit of lifting them up. When we choose to do these things, we are keeping happiness in the front of our minds as often as we can, which leads to the creation of a happy life.

Choose Laughter over Annoyance

You can't take life too seriously.
You just have to laugh your way through it.
—Marjorie Pay Hinckley

So many of our experiences in life can be miserable, annoying, and frustrating. But if we can choose to look at these stumbling blocks with humor and the absurdity that they often deserve, they can turn bad days into good ones, and aggravating times into happy and funny memories. It's a conscious choice to look at things one way over another, and most of the times, laughter is the best way to flip the switch from exasperating to comical.

When we moved my daughter out of her apartment upon graduating from college, we found ourselves unable to release her bike from the rack due to a rusted and therefore impenetrable lock. After optimistically (but ultimately unsuccessfully) attempting to cut through the spiral part of the lock with the tools at our disposal—tin snips, a branch lopper, and portable jigsaw left at our house by the previous owners—we realized that we had to go to the hardware store to get a stronger implement that would do the job.

After going up and down the same two aisles multiple times, we finally located the bolt cutters we would need (and we also picked up a hand saw, just in case), ran back under the now rainy skies to free the bike from its shackled state, and our efforts were rewarded by a giant glorious rainbow greeting us out the windows on our way home.

Throughout the afternoon—as a thirty-second task ended up taking the better part of two hours—we could have chosen to be annoyed and frustrated, and then more angry and irritated with each obstacle. When each tool didn't work, we giggled, especially when the blade flew off of the jigsaw. When we realized that we would have trouble explaining ourselves if law enforcement had happened by, as we looked like the loudest, most ineffective bike thieves ever, we were doubled over with laughter. When we couldn't find what we needed in the store despite our best hunting efforts, we cracked each other up talking about the funny ways we might use other tools instead. Then when the rain started—of course it started raining—we chose to see the absurdity of it all and laughed through our ultimate triumphant moment. But aren't there people that you know who would have taken each setback as an opportunity to get more frustrated and upset?

It also never entered our minds to give up on the situation, no matter how difficult it became. We knew that we would be able to figure out a solution, no matter how many tries it took, and I think that is a really important lesson for when we're faced with seemingly insurmountable things in our lives. When we set our minds to "I CAN do this" and "I WILL do this," then it becomes a matter of just finding the right way to do it, and never "this is too hard" or "this is impossible."

We never know what hurdles or stumbling blocks life is going to throw at us. Oftentimes we cannot control the hardships and misfortunes that may come our way. But we **can** control how we deal with them. Choosing laughter over annoyance isn't always easy, but it starts with a mindset of keeping things in perspective and consciously deciding how we are going to react to them.

A few questions to consider:

Has being angry or bothered by things outside of our control EVER made them better?

Has choosing to be irritated and annoyed by minor inconveniences EVER made someone's life better or more satisfying?

Has seeing the bright side of a situation and laughing through difficulty EVER had a downside to someone's daily existence?

There are people who will try to tell you that being happy is a waste of time because life will always disappoint you. These same people will go through their lives being proud of their misery and holding it up for everyone to see. They will take every opportunity to see the bad in situations, blame others and the outside world for their woes, and make the choice to get angry at the hard things rather than laugh at them.

They don't feel like it's a choice, but it is. It actually is. And we have the power to make that choice in every moment of our lives. Which will you choose?

Happiness Teflon

As much as I try to not allow the mean things that mean people say to affect me, recently someone was very nasty to me, and it made me really upset.

For two days.

I'm not sure why it affected me this much, but on the evening of the second day as I was standing at the sink washing the dishes, I kept turning it over and over in my mind, all the while wishing I could just let it go and not have it bother me anymore.

At one point as I was putting something onto the drying rack I spotted our one remaining non-stick Teflon* pan.

In seeing it I kind of marveled at its ability to not have anything stick to it, and if something does, it's so easily washed away.

I wondered in that moment, if it would be possible to cover myself in metaphorical Teflon, so that things—especially ones that stay on and burn—wouldn't stick.

How's that for a concept? Could we be the embodiment of the old "I'm rubber and you're glue, anything you say bounces off of me and sticks to you" response to a bully on the playground?

---

*I am fully aware of the controversy surrounding the use of Teflon cookware and its potential toxicity. We only have one pan, and it's only used about four times a year when my husband makes crepes.

As I kept thinking about it, I realized that I had already experienced this a few times, and I needed to acknowledge how strong and powerful wearing Teflon armor can be.

A few years ago, while I was driving, I was going down a hill toward a traffic light at the bottom. I was just calmly going along, minding the speed limit, listening to the radio, when out of nowhere a car came tearing up behind me and riding my tail the rest of the way down the hill.

There was nowhere for me to go, no other lane to get into, and within a few seconds the driver had sped around me to get to the left turning lane at the traffic light. Just as he arrived there, the left arrow light that had been yellow, turned red, and he was stuck there, unable to go any further.

Meanwhile, I was still going the same regular speed, nearly at the bottom of the hill, and as I was about to go through the green light that was approaching in my lane, I saw the driver unbuckle his seat belt, move over to the passenger side of the car, put down that window, and proceed to "flip me the bird" out the window just as I passed by.

I'm sure he was hoping that I would be upset or hurt by his rude gesture, but I honestly found it hilarious. The fact that he would take all of that time and trouble to undo his seat belt, move all the way over, and do what he did, just for the express purpose of making sure I knew just how angry he was, made me laugh at how utterly important it was to this guy to blame me for his current situation.

Despite his intention, I was not upset at all. In my previous "people-pleasing" days I would have been distraught and remorseful because I had inadvertently caused a complete stranger frustration and anger, and I would have subjected myself to these bad feelings because I believed that feeling the way they wanted me to feel was necessary. But now I realize that **I do not have any responsibility whatsoever to feel a certain way simply because someone else wants me to.** *Furthermore, why should someone else's feelings have more importance or validity than mine?*

Now, if I have hurt or disappointed someone I will absolutely apologize in earnest and try to do whatever I can to make up for the detriment I have caused. But if a complete stranger decides to take offense for something that I unintentionally did or said, then I have no obligation whatsoever to feel badly about it. I have that choice to make, especially when I am trying to make healthy choices about what I allow to enter my psyche and, more importantly, what I don't.

So when someone is mean to you, think of yourself coated in Happiness Teflon. Have what they say or do bounce right off of you, and most likely it will land back on them because P.S. that's how karma works.

Practice Optimism

Optimist: Someone who figures that taking
a step backward after taking a step forward
isn't a disaster, it's a cha-cha.
—Robert Brault

I know a lot of pessimistic people. They are convinced that if they look forward to something they will ultimately be disappointed, and they also believe that the very act of being optimistic will actually *cause* the other proverbial shoe to drop.

Question: When was the last time that simply thinking one way or another about something changed the actual outcome? Oh that's right, NEVER.

Just the same as worrying has never once made a difference in how something was going to ultimately turn out, "not worrying," or choosing to be excited and optimistic about something, also does not have any bearing on how something is going to happen. But being optimistic and looking forward to things DOES have a huge effect on our reality BEFORE it happens, and that effect can make our life a lovely, happy, and uplifting place to be.

Something important to remember about optimism is that it's easy to do when things are entirely within our control. Take planning a trip: When we get to the special event or vacation, most of what happens there can be completely *out* of our control. Things like bad weather, a shortage of restaurant staff, unclean hotel rooms, and other unforeseen circumstances can really put a damper on what was supposed to be a great time that we had looked forward to. But let me be the one to tell you this: **These unfortunate things were going to happen whether you worried about them happening, whether you didn't even think about them happening, or whether you fully expected them NOT to happen.** Therefore, you might as well enjoy the time leading up to the special event because then you at least had some happiness and excitement in your everyday life as you looked forward to something that was going to be potentially wonderful and tremendous and beautiful.

You cannot cause anything bad to happen by being happy about it beforehand, and you cannot prevent bad things from happening by worrying about them ahead of time. Period. End of story.

As mentioned in "Always Have Something to Look Forward To," having that next thing or things to anticipate with joy and enthusiasm can often make the difference between a happy life and an unhappy one.

And if the thing that you were looking forward to ends up disappointing you, well then you can chalk that up to "this is how things turn out sometimes" and move on to the next thing. Disappointment is never a reason to give up hope for something better around the corner, and just because one thing didn't turn out the way you expected is no guarantee that the next thing will have the same result.

Many people fall into this trap—with relationships, with jobs, with all aspects of their lives. They believe that since the last person they grew close to hurt them, the next person will too, as will the person after that, and so on and so on. Lots of people think that because they had a few jobs that were unfulfilling or discouraging, all jobs henceforth will be similar. It's very easy to remain pessimistic and sour toward the really important things in our lives, so that we avoid being disappointed in the future. But I, for one, would rather have weeks and months of joy leading up to something, followed by a possible disappointment (that would inevitably be shorter than the "looking forward to it" time), than have all of that time being miserable and negative while I expected things to fall short of my expectations. Yes, it kind of prevents us from disappointment, but it also prevents us from living our lives as happily as possible.

> *Optimism is the faith that leads to achievement.*
> *Nothing can be done without hope and confidence.*
> —Helen Keller

Without optimism, we have no faith. Without optimism, we have no hope. Without optimism, we have no joy.

Choose to be optimistic and make it a practice in your life. Always always always have something to look forward to, and spend your energy looking forward to it. You won't regret it, no matter how the thing you optimistically anticipated turns out, I promise.

Happiness Tools in Your Toolbox

We've all heard about having the right metaphorical tools in our metaphorical toolboxes to help us handle any situation. We try to raise our kids with confidence tactics, coping skills, and time management expertise so when they enter the real world they will be able to handle whatever life throws at them.

But how often do we think about a toolbox for happiness? What are some things that we can curate and draw upon when we're faced with a situation that is bringing us the opposite of joy? How can we consciously combat things like sadness, frustration, anger, resentment, and annoyance, to help keep us on the track to choosing happiness in those difficult times?

After doing some research and asking people to describe their own happiness toolboxes, I have developed a toolbox of my own that I recently had to open up when I was dealing with a less-than-ideal situation from which I was physically unable to remove myself. Some of them may seem silly or goofy, but as long as they work, who cares? It's up to each of us to define and gather the set of tools that works best for whatever we might be going through.

1. **Music.** I have a list of "Happy Songs" that I consciously listen to that helps me to get myself out of a funk. I also have nostalgic songs that remind me of hopeful

times, and I have songs that make me feel powerful and strong. Music is a very important tool for me, and it can have a magical effect on our mood and our psyche. (More on this in "Music Is Magic.") Try experimenting with different genres and artists you may not be familiar with. You never know what is going to affect you in a positive way, so keep those ears open and keep the music flowing as you're choosing healthy and happy thoughts and actions in your life.

2. **Smiling.** I talk about this a lot. When you're in a tough spot, forcing yourself to smile, and even laughing if you're able to, tricks your brain into thinking you're happy. Once your brain starts releasing those happy chemicals, the bad mood dissipates, and before you know it, you're in a much better place mentally than you were before.

3. **Ribbons in my hair.** I know this might sound ridiculous for a grown woman, but I cannot be negative or sullen when I have some bright ribbons in my hair. I will often tie on ribbons when we're cheering for our team in the Super Bowl or while watching the Olympics, and this simple little act always brightens my spirits and puts me in a celebratory mood. I have been known to put colorful ribbons in my hair even when there's not a big sports event going on, because it's an easy and tangible thing I can do to keep my own little corner of the world festive and cheery.

Similar to this theme, I know a fellow mom who has a tiara that she proudly wears when she's folding laundry or doing chores around the house. It reminds her that no matter what she's doing, she's a queen who's in charge and has the crown to prove it.

4. **Games, Table Topics Questions, Coloring Books and Crayons, etc.** I remember a time when I would never bring my kids to a restaurant or an airplane or another such place where sitting still for a long period of time was required without a bag filled with books and toys and activities to keep them occupied. Talk about having a necessary toolbox! I have found that the same approach works with grown-ups, especially with people that you don't know well or even whom you might not particularly like. I was recently in that very situation, and although I was absolutely dreading it, I came armed with fun discussion topics, a big bag filled with board games, and a book of interesting and unique "Mind Bender" questions. Sure enough, there were multiple times when all of us were required to be in the same room with nothing to do, and there was even a time when a group activity became unexpectedly postponed and we were all stuck for two hours in a rather confined space. Yikes! As you might imagine, patience began to run low and tempers began to run high. Luckily, I had tools in my toolbox, and I started bringing out the questions and the games and encouraged everyone to join in. Almost immediately frowns turned into smiles, irritations cooled off, and we found ourselves laughing and acting out silly things and enjoying this unexpected time together. What started out as a difficult situation became a fun and engaging one instead. Sometimes all you need is a little forethought and preparation, and those tools can make all the difference.

5. **Language.** Have an Encouragement Box, Jar, or Book filled with funny and encouraging quotes to draw upon when you need a pick-me-up. (P.S. This makes a great gift for someone who is going through a rough patch.)

These are just a few ideas for your own happiness toolbox. Everything in life is better when we are as prepared as possible, and for those unexpected twists and turns that could easily take us off of our choosing happiness path, we have to have the tools we need to keep us healthily on track. And whatever works for you is perfectly fine; it doesn't matter what anyone else thinks about it. A plumber can't do his or her job without the right wrenches and pipe snakes, a carpenter can't do his or her job without the right hammers and saws, a doctor can't do his or her job without the right stethoscope, medicines, etc., and we can't do our jobs of living the best and happiest lives we possibly can without the right tools either. Figure out what they are, pack your toolbox full, and you'll be ready to handle any situation that isn't inherently happy for yourself.

Happiness is a choice that requires effort at times.
—Aeschylus

Sharpen those happiness tools and use them!

Don't Complain

There's a famous story about Dolly Parton that I love. It goes that while she and her fellow actresses were shooting the film *Steel Magnolias* there was a Christmastime scene taking place on an outside porch and everyone was bundled up in wool sweaters and coats. Unfortunately, they were shooting in the middle of the summer in the sweltering heat and humidity of Louisiana. There was an especially long wait to begin filming and everyone started complaining about how hot they were in their costumes. Everyone except Dolly Parton, who was delightedly singing to herself while she swung blissfully on a nearby tree swing. At one point one of the actresses went over to her and asked something like, "Dolly, aren't you dying of the heat? It's soooo hot in these sweaters and we've been waiting for such a long time…" and Dolly looked at her and said sweetly, "All my life I've wanted to be a movie star and I ain't about to complain about what comes with it."

That silenced the young ingénue immediately. I adore this story because it is such a perfect example of recognizing the good in a situation and realizing that in just about every scenario you can choose to look at the good part of it or focus your energy on the bad part of it. We always have that choice, just as Dolly did.

There's another quote that I love, from Laura Ingalls Wilder. She said, "We have a slight headache and we mention the fact. As an excuse to ourselves for inflicting it upon our friends we make it as bad as possible in the telling. 'Oh I have such a dreadful headache,' we say and we immediately feel much worse. Our pain has grown from the talking of it. If we have a headache, we will forget it sooner if we talk of pleasant things."

Haven't you found this to be true? When we're complaining about something, doesn't the issue we're complaining about instantly get exponentially worse? And what good does complaining do anyway? It never actually improves the situation or makes us feel any better about it.

I think the reason we like to complain is to somehow show the situation that it doesn't have power over us, or to show ourselves that despite what we're dealing with, we still have the upper hand. But wouldn't choosing joy or contentment or the resolution to wait out the bad thing while keeping our spirits up be better ways of exerting whatever control over it that we can?

When I was in college, I became very friendly with a girl who complained all the time. Everything was miserable, everything had a bad side, and I found myself getting caught up in her negativity. It was kind of fun actually, at the time, to grumble about things and turn a cynical eye on everything around us. We became inseparable, and while I didn't feel like I was turning into a negative, grouchy, somewhat sullen person, other people took notice of the change in me, and very kindly let me know.

After a few months, one friend took me aside and said, in the kindest way possible, "You know, you're not the same Rachel that I really enjoyed meeting and spending time with when you first came here. I think it's because you're hanging out with so-and-so all the time." I was very surprised to hear this, and this friend went on to say, "I really miss that person because she was so happy and optimistic and friendly, and I don't want to see you disappear down this dark road instead."

These comments hurt my feelings, and even after taking a long hard look at myself, I decided that having this friend was more important that what I was turning into, so we got even closer and ended up becoming roommates. We had a grand old time griping about every little thing and talking about people behind their backs, all the while feeling terribly superior to everyone else.

Then came another comment, this one from the friend's brand new boyfriend (who, by the way, would shortly thereafter go on to break her heart so severely that she did something so horrible it caused her to move out, us to sever ties completely, and we never spoke to each other again).

What he said to me was, "Jeez Rachel, you wouldn't know what to come out of your mouth if it wasn't complaining about something."

Can I be honest? Even after all of these years, that comment still stings. It hurt me tremendously at the time, and he was clearly a jerk on so many levels, but truthfully it was one of those moments where somebody in my life said the exact right thing to me that I needed to hear at the exact right time. I felt like I had been punched squarely in the gut—and it was precisely what I needed to help me get my life back on track. Shortly after that, when the friend and I stopped speaking, and after the darkness of the cruelty and the betrayal passed, it was like the sun came out on my life and I never looked back.

I learned a vital life lesson from that experience, and as a result I make the choice to refrain from complaining as much as humanly possible. I always try to see the silver lining, and when I do choose to vent about things that are frustrating or irritating or downright maddening, I make sure to get it out of my system quickly and move on.

To that point, I do believe that there is a time and a place for blowing off steam and not letting bad things get bottled up inside you. But it's also important in those times to have a clear intention and to not let the complaining take over the overall joy and peace you are cultivating in your daily life.

The late Randy Pausch put it best in his book *The Last Lecture* when he said, "You have to decide if you're going to be a Tigger or an Eeyore." Well, I have been the Eeyore, and I can tell you, being a Tigger is a better way to live.

Despite what some people may think, you don't get any mythical points in life for suffering the most or for letting everyone else know, in great detail, what's wrong with you or what is currently troubling you at the moment. What you DO get out of life is the opportunity to make it as happy and joyful and productive and fulfilling as you can. So make the choice to NOT complain. The more we complain, the more unhappy we get.

Happiness is letting go of what you think
your life is supposed to look like and
celebrating it for everything that it is.

—MINDY HALE

If You Want to Feel Sorry for Yourself, Set a Timer

There's a great line in the movie *Sixteen Candles*. Samantha is upset because her family forgot about her sixteenth birthday, and her best friend says to her, "Would you stop feeling sorry for yourself! It's bad for your complexion!"

I love that! It's so true too. It's also bad for our minds, our souls, our bodies, and our personal growth.

However, I will add to this that at times it's necessary to feel sorry for ourselves and acknowledging what's wrong can sometimes provide us with some benefit. How? It must be done consciously, purposefully, and above all, in moderation.

I read that after Christopher Reeve's paralyzing accident he allowed himself twenty minutes every morning to cry and acknowledge his unthinkable situation. He noted how important that time was for him, allowing himself to feel the intense loss and the challenges he was facing, so that he could *consciously make the shift* to feeling hopeful and optimistic. Because he gave himself permission to recognize and feel the bad stuff, he was able to then put it away and focus on the good.

This is not easy to do. It's much easier to sit in the mire of our discontent or frustration and tell ourselves that we deserve to feel this way. We can feel righteously entitled to pity ourselves for what happened to us, and we can get into an unhealthy pattern of focusing on how rotten things are and what a shame it is that we've been hurt, disappointed, or discouraged. Those feelings can be very comfortable for a lot of us, and it can be difficult to pull ourselves out of that ever-darkening hole of despair and misery.

But ask yourself, do you really want to live that way? Do you want your life to be you essentially walking around with your chin in your hands saying "Poor me" all the time?

If not, then you have to **make the choice** to feel those feelings, acknowledge them for what they are and their presence in your life, and then **put them away** to make room for hope and happiness.

Because it can be so hard to get ourselves out of what feels comfortable and safe, I suggest using a timer for your self-pity sessions. Set the timer for 5, 10, 15, 20 minutes—however long you think you'll need that day—and then go for it! Cry, scream, punch a pillow, throw things (soft things that won't hurt you or your surroundings), do whatever it is that you need to do to get the bad feelings out of yourself. When the timer goes off, dry your tears, wash your face, put the pillows back where they belong, and get on with your day.

It really works! Acknowledging pain, both mental and physical, gives it less power over us and allows us to recognize it for where it stands in the grand scheme of our lives. This exercise can also show us that whatever the difficult thing is, it is NOT stronger than we are. It can be a purposeful way to take control over our misery and remind it who's boss.

So while it seems counterintuitive, I'm actually in favor of feeling sorry for ourselves sometimes. But set a timer, and when the time is up, leave the unhappiness where it is and move on. Your mind, your body, your spirit, and yes, your complexion, will thank you.

Don't Save Anything for a Special Occasion

Being alive is the special occasion.

I recently had the opportunity and honor to help in cleaning out my husband's grandmother's house after her death at ninety-five years old. She had lived in the house for nearly seventy years, and while she wasn't a materialistic person, there was still quite an accumulation of "stuff" that naturally builds up when you raise six kids and several grandchildren in the same place for so long.

Along with the bookshelves filled with books and closets full of clothes and linens, I was stunned by the mountains of dishes and crockery and mugs and vases that were spread out on several tables for people to go through and tag if they wanted to take them home as a remembrance of Grandma. While a few things were selected because of sentimental value, we spent the rest of the afternoon packing up the rest to go to Goodwill or into the pile for the dump run.

As I observed this whole process, what struck me was that the things that were once fundamental parts of a person's life were now trash. As I wrapped up countless "free giveaway" glasses and commemorative ceramic spoon rests, one thought kept going through my mind:

Use what you have NOW and get rid of the rest.

Because we have moved across the country a few times, my family doesn't have a ton of nonessential things taking up space in our home. But after I got back from the trip and assessed the boxes of "good dishes" that we rarely use, and the random once-used appliances that were well-intentioned gifts, I decided that there is no point in saving anything for another time or a special occasion—the time to use these things is NOW. If there's anything that I discover I don't want to use, then I really shouldn't save it for someone else to have to get rid of later. If one person's trash is another person's treasure, then the reverse is also most certainly true.

I knew someone who had a set of crystal glasses that she kept way up high in a nearly inaccessible cabinet in her dining room. Once I was helping her set the table for a dinner party and she was bemoaning her lack of matching wine glasses. "Why don't you use those ones up there?" I asked, gesturing up to the fancy goblets.

"Oh no," she answered. "I can't use those."

"Why not?" I asked.

"Because," she answered, "They don't make that pattern anymore, so if one of them breaks I can't get a replacement."

This response baffled me. I remember thinking to myself (but refrained from saying out loud), "What a pessimistic way of looking at things. You're assuming the worst and expecting calamity to occur. Why would you rob yourself of enjoying something that you cherish, just because there is an infinitesimal and highly unlikely chance that something bad will happen?" Then I thought about the fact that if something was designed for a particular use, doesn't it make sense to use it for the purpose for which it was made? I remember thinking the same thing when I asked that same friend when we were younger if we could play with the dolls she had up on her bedroom shelf. She responded curtly, "These dolls aren't for playing with, they are for display." And even at that age I remember thinking to myself, "They make dolls for DISPLAY? It's a doll! It's meant to be played with!"

Clearly I've never been a "For Display Only" type of person. I let my daughter wear her flower girl dress to preschool every day because I knew that all too soon she would grow out of it. I let my son wear my grandfather's antique ring when he wanted to rather than have it sit in a dusty box in a drawer. I allowed both of my kids to take the tags off of their Beanie Babies and throw them around the room playing Stuffed Animal Olympics rather than keep them in pristine condition in case they were worth something someday.

At the end of the day, and especially at the end of someone's life, things are just things. Teacups get broken, curtains fade in the sun, beloved books get dog-eared, and favorite pens run out of ink. Yes, things should be valued and treated with respect, but they should also be used while we are still living and breathing and have the chance to receive the pleasure they were designed to give.

So my advice for choosing happiness to you is this: Use the pretty glasses and don't worry if one of them might break. Wear the special shirt you bought because you loved it instead of letting it sit in your closet because you're worried about the possibility of spilling coffee on it. Break out the pasta machine or the Belgian waffle maker once in a while and treat your family to something different from the regular old fare that you're all used to. Use your things or let them go so someone else can use them and experience the joy for which they were originally intended.

Don't ever save anything for a special occasion. Being alive is indeed the most special occasion there is.

Set Healthy Boundaries for Yourself

When we're trying to choose happiness in our lives that can often mean letting go of what we think is expected of us in order for us to truly be happy. I can't remember where I first heard this sentence, but I love it:

Always remember that "No." is a complete sentence.

N.O. Period.

You don't have to give excuses or reasons for saying "No," all you have to do is say it, and then say it again if someone isn't taking your "No" for an answer.

No one's time is more important than yours, and you have permission to say an emphatic "No" to the things that don't keep you on your road toward happiness in your life. It may be a tough choice to make sometimes, but that one little word could open up a bevy of opportunity for things to say an enthusiastic "Yes!" to instead.

Say Yes to Things!

While it is vitally important to say "No" to things and people that don't help us achieve our goals, it is equally important to say a whole-hearted "Yes" to as many things as possible. Life presents us with so many opportunities every single day, and if we're too busy looking down at our phones or binge-watching TV or resting comfortably in our fears of trying something new, we will undoubtedly miss out on countless chances for joy and fun and excitement. Who doesn't need more of those things in their daily lives?

I recently devoured *Year of Yes* by Shonda Rhimes. In it she describes her experiment of consciously saying "Yes" to anything and everything that scared her, and when her young children asked her to drop everything and play with them.

She made the commitment for a full year, and she honored it. Even on her way out to an awards show, dressed up in a formal gown and diamond earrings, when her daughter asked her to get down on the floor and play, Shonda did just that. It was only for ten minutes, but she made sure to stay true to what she promised herself, and in doing so, her daughter knew that she was just as important to her mommy as her work engagement.

She also said "Yes" to invitations from friends and colleagues, to vacation get-aways that she had always meant to take, along with speaking engagements and production meetings for new shows she had previously been too afraid or self-conscious to present.

The impetus for this drastic switch-up in her daily existence came because her sister said to her multi-award winning, incredibly groundbreaking, glass ceiling shattering, phenomenally successful younger sister (Shonda), "You never say yes to anything."

That was a pivotal moment in Shonda's life because she realized that with all of her accolades and acclaim, she was also missing out on so many other things that could bring her fulfillment and joy. Especially when it came to her kids.

It made me wonder how much we miss out on when we instinctively say "No" because we feel like we're too busy or too stressed or have too much else going on. I also wonder how much we disappoint other people when we choose to say no to what they offer us, which is an easy thing to miss when all we're thinking about is ourselves.

Which made me think of shoo-fly pie.*

One day when I was about eleven or twelve, a friend of mine's family took me to a county fair that they attended every year. It was your typical outdoor event with pony rides, livestock shows, and carnival rides. Shortly after we arrived, we stopped at a huge table filled with baked goods for sale. My friend got a piece of shoo-fly pie and her eyes lit up as the man behind the counter handed it to her. My mouth started watering just looking at it (I had never had shoo-fly

---

*Shoo-fly pie is a Pennsylvania Dutch confection reminiscent of pecan pie without the pecans. I recommend it highly.

pie before, but it looked amazing). Her mom kindly asked me, "Rachel, would you like a slice?" Every vibrating molecule of me wanted to say, "Yes, please," but instead I remembered that under no circumstances was I to be any kind of burden to anyone, financially or otherwise, and so I slowly shook my head and replied forlornly, "No, thanks." The mom looked at me and asked again, "Are you sure? You are welcome to get whatever you want." I looked longingly at that big table filled with delicious looking confections and considered saying "Yes" for about a full second, then once again remembered what I believed to be "my place" and said, as convincingly as I could, "No, thanks, I'm good."

Looking back on this scene now I realize that not only did I let my own distorted feelings about my self-worth rob me of a happy moment (and a very tasty piece of pie), but I also deprived my friend's mom of the chance to show me a good time and do what she could to make sure I was enjoying myself. It didn't occur to me then, or even until recently, that me saying "No" was denying someone else the pleasure and joy of showing kindness.

This reminds me of what a friend of mine told me about her mother making sure to say "Yes" to people after her husband passed away. She knew that when someone repeatedly says "No" to offers of getting together, at some point the offers stop coming. So even though there were many times when she would have rather just stayed inside, simmering in her grief, she accepted all of her friends' invitations, knowing that the sadness would still be there at home for her when she returned.

This is not to say that a person needs to put on a brave face and ignore their feelings in order to satisfy another person's desire for them to do so. But it's just a gentle encouragement for all of us to remember that saying "Yes," even when we might not want to, can bring us out of our own heads and provide us a door to happiness we didn't know was waiting for us to open.

Replace "I Have to" with "I Choose to," or Even Better, "I Get To"

Some years ago, I was complaining about having to do something I really didn't want to do. I can't remember what it was, but I remember how my friend replied to my grumbling.

She said, "I used to complain about that kind of stuff. Now instead of saying "I HAVE to," I say "I CHOOSE to.""

Whoa. What a concept. Not only does it give me emotional power over the situation, but it also changes it from a burden to an opportunity.

How cool is that? The thing we have to do remains the same, but our mindset can completely flip it from negative to positive.

Brilliant.

Seems simple, but that doesn't make it easy.

Here's an example of this in practice: I used to dread cleaning my house. (I'm not one of those people who gets excited about cleaning, and honestly, I'm a little envious of those people sometimes.) I would procrastinate and usually only get around to it when it became absolutely necessary. But once I tried flipping it around in my brain, I realized that if I was making the choice to do it, it would bring me so much satisfaction, and if I was realizing how lucky I was to "get" to do this thing, it could actually bring me joy.

So there I was, bucket of cleaning supplies in hand, going around and saying things like, "I'm choosing to do this so my family and I can live comfortably and healthily in a dust-free, clutter-free, peaceful home." And, "I'm making this choice so we can all relax later and not have to worry about the dishes in the sink or what is building up in the corners of the shower."

Then I also started thinking, "This is actually pretty great. This is some nice 'me' time, where I don't have to think about work, where no one else is taking away my attention, and I can actually see the results of my labor, which are quite satisfying!"

It happily snowballed from there. As I kept moving through the house, I thought things such as "While I'm scrubbing this toilet, I can realize how lucky I am to have running water and working pipes and that there are actually two toilets in this house for four people." And, "While I'm cleaning these kitchen appliances, I can remember how grateful I am to have an oven large enough to fit a turkey, as my first three living spaces did not." There's nothing like appreciating the fact that you have a house to clean that meets the needs of your family to turn the task into an actual act of gratitude.

Here's another example: No one likes going to places where you know you'll be stuck in a long line, like the DMV, the post office, crowded big box stores, and places like that. I used to dread that tedium as well, but now I turn those waiting times into opportunities for fun. If my kids are with me, we'll play those car games like "Alphabet" or "I Spy" or one of our all-time favorites, which we call "What's He/She

Thinking?" where we whisper to each other what the people around us might be thinking based on their expressions and body language.

If I'm by myself, I resist the urge to pull out my phone, and instead allow myself to daydream about things like a new place I'd like to visit, a creative project I'd like to tackle, or something interesting I'm going to cook next. I will sometimes play word games on my phone if the line is really long, but those are good for my brain synapses, and they're a conscious choice I can make that allows me to focus on something other than the fact that I've been standing in the same place for so long with no discernible signs of when my turn will finally come up.

One more example, and this is perhaps the hardest one because it involves dealing with other people. There are times when we have no choice but to spend time with people whom we'd rather not. I struggle with finding the "I choose to" in these situations because I would honestly rather NOT choose to, and I certainly would not consider it something that I gladly "get to" do. In these cases, I go to gratitude and tell myself things like this:

"At least it's not worse. It may be bad, but it could be worse." (Because things could *always* be worse.)

"This is just for now, it's not forever."

If a meal is involved, I can focus on being grateful for the food and say to myself, "Yum, this is delicious! If I wasn't here, I wouldn't have the chance to have this wonderful food."

If I'm outside I can focus on the nature around me and be grateful for the fresh air I'm breathing, the colors I'm seeing, and the sounds I'm hearing. In those times I say to myself, "I'm so glad to have the chance to be outside and experience my current landscape in this way."

The point is, we all have to do things that we don't want to do. But when we're consciously choosing happiness, we can make the choice of how we deal with them while they're going on. Change "I have to" to "I choose to" or "I get to."

(And if all else fails, just be sure to be grateful when the situation is over and move on with your joyful life.)

Remove Yourself
from the Situation

Even if that situation is just in your own mind.

We've all been in circumstances where we can feel our tempers rising due to annoyance or anger, or the beginning of an emotional downturn into sadness and despair. In those times it's so important that we recognize what's going on, and when possible, to physically remove ourselves from that location to prevent an irate outburst or a dark spiral into our own despondence. I strongly encourage you to make the choice to get out of that space whenever possible, to preserve your own sanity and inner peace.

But what about for those times when we can't remove ourselves? When physically leaving would cause more problems down the line that we do not want to have to deal with? One suggestion would be to remove yourself from the situation mentally.

In your mind, take yourself to a happy place (see "Find Your Happy Place") and consciously imagine yourself being there. Try closing your eyes and really immersing yourself in the sights and sounds and smells of that place. Sometimes you only need a few seconds of this mental vacation to instill within yourself the calmness and serenity needed to withstand the current situation.

Another way to remove yourself mentally is to consciously feel the soles of your feet attached to where they are and "ground yourself." When you do this, you remind yourself of your own strength and that you have the power to not get caught up in the outer nonsense. Planting your feet and feeling them firmly attached to the floor or ground or wherever you are standing or sitting is an effective and unobtrusive way to perceptually get yourself out of a harried or stressful situation. (It can be especially great to do at work, especially during a difficult or marathonic meeting.)

Sometimes we get into situations that are completely caused by ourselves and our own thoughts. Oftentimes while we're just going along in our day, our thoughts can be triggered by things we see or memories that pop up, and we find ourselves in a state of anger or melancholy as a result. What do we do then?

In those instances, I would advise:

Remove yourself from yourself.

What does this mean? Well, we can do the same things that we do when removing ourselves from situations that involve other people. For example, maybe you're in the kitchen chopping vegetables and out of the blue a thought comes in or you're reminded of something that makes you upset. When this happens, immediately remove yourself from where you are standing and force your brain to move on to wherever you are going and whatever new thing you are going to do. If you stay in the physical spot where the trigger happened, your mind could get stuck in an endless loop of thinking about it and ruminating over it and turning it over and over in your mind. You will most likely end up becoming more and more agitated or distraught about it—so make the choice to deliberately break free from it. Put down the knife, leave the kitchen, and go somewhere else purposefully. Maybe go outside and get the mail. Maybe grab the dog and go for a walk. Maybe go upstairs to change the sheets on the bed. Whatever it is, **remove yourself from yourself**. Snapping the brain out of its entrenched circuitry can be very powerful and helpful when it tries to take over and repeat old thought patterns of self-destruction and misery.

When we realize that we are doing this to ourselves we also realize that we can STOP doing it to ourselves. We always have the power to change our thoughts, and in doing so, we can healthily alter the mental space we're living in and how we feel about that space at any moment.

If we're making happiness a choice in our daily lives then we need to be hyper-cognizant of where our minds are and how the voices in our minds can affect us. The more we practice removing ourselves and focusing on something else when our thoughts are negative and stress-inducing, the less we will find ourselves having to do so.

Create Your Own Community of People Who Lift You Up

And banish the ones who don't.

Ok, that seems harsh. Instead let's just say "let go" of the ones who don't.

Have the right people around you is essential when you are choosing happiness in your life. Much like we cull material things when we de-clutter our physical spaces, it's vitally important that we make deliberate choices about with whom we are going to spend time in those places. Having friends and family members who encourage you and bring you up when you're feeling down is an essential part of happiness, and too often we allow the wrong people to influence our decisions and keep us stuck in a miserable place we'd rather not inhabit.

It can be very difficult to let go of people in our lives, especially when they've been with us for a long time. But like when we're discarding material things, we ask ourselves, "Does this item still serve the goals and aspirations I have now, and want for my future?" If the answer is "no," then we let it go. The same has to be done for people who are not sharing our same vision.

It is not selfish to take care of yourself by surrounding yourself with only the people that support you and encourage you. I cannot stress this enough. The people whom you allow into your world can be extremely instrumental in the kind of life that you choose to have. If there are people who may not be meeting your expectations in the friend department, then I would ask yourself these questions:

For someone you've been friends with for a long time:

If I met this person now, would I want to be friends with them, or would I turn and run away as quickly as possible?

When I talk with this person, do they constantly bring up the past and relive old memories because it's all we have in common anymore?

Does this person still treat me the same way as when we were younger, and if so, have I moved on from being that person and would prefer to be treated differently?

Does this person fit into my current definition of what is a "friend," or are they still around simply because they have been for so long?

I'm not saying that it's not incredibly wonderful to have old good friends. People who know all about us and were there for us for the big moments as well as the small, seemingly insignificant times are treasures, and if you are lucky enough to have old friends who have grown with you through the years then that is a blessing beyond measure. But if you have old friends who, like clothing styles and toy fads, no longer fit into the life you want for yourself, then maybe it's time to reevaluate their presence in your life.

You don't necessarily have to ban them from your existence. This can be nearly impossible, especially if you live near each other and frequent the same neighborhood places. But I would encourage you to perhaps "demote" them, at least in your mind, to a lower level of friendship, like say, an acquaintance.

It has been vitally helpful for me to have different categories of friends throughout my life. They have changed with time, but some of the titles have been:

Best Friends, Good Friends, Good Acquaintances, Acquaintances, and the People I've Recently Met Who May Fit into One of Those Categories at Some Point.

I've had people move between the categories—a Good Acquaintance who became a Good Friend, a Best Friend who became an Acquaintance, and everything in-between, depending on what was going on in our lives. Friend relationships can have a healthy fluidity, as long as you both have the same expectations of being the kind of friend that each other needs you to be.

I know a lot of people who are afraid to let go of people because they are afraid of being lonely or because they believe a bad friend is better than no friend at all. To this I would say that while being alone is hard, being with someone who constantly puts you down and doesn't support you is far worse. You have your own definitions of what a good friend, a friend, or an acquaintance needs to be for you, and if a person isn't meeting those requirements, then much like in an employer/employee environment, you have every right to let them go in order to make room for someone else who will serve in that position more effectively.

To that point, you should never keep someone in your life just because you don't think you will meet other people. There are tons of ways to make new acquaintances and friends, including:

Join a Meetup group for something that you enjoy doing and you will meet other similarly-minded people there with whom you already have something important in common.

Strike up a conversation with someone at the gym. It's not as hard as you might think. Ask someone for a spot if you're lifting weights or make a commiserating comment to someone about how hot it is in the room or how early in the morning it is.

Try the same thing at the grocery store. If you're standing next to someone and you're both looking at the apples, try saying something like, "There are so many choices, I don't know which one to pick—what's your favorite kind?" It's the same advice we were taught about making friends as kids: Put yourself out there and try connecting with someone else. It may work, it may not, but you never know until you try.

Take a class in something that you either already like or would like to try. Cooking, yoga, pottery, acting, Jiu Jitsu, knitting, photography, guitar, bowling, woodworking, glassblowing, the list is truly endless. While you're there, consciously engage with the people around you whenever possible. Compliment someone on how they are doing and encourage them as they go. You are all already in a collective vulnerable state by putting yourselves out there to do this thing, which can provide a leveling comfort to help you support one another.

Something else to remember about the people you meet is that many of them were only meant to be a part of your life for a season. I have many fond memories of friends I had for certain times in my life, and then we drifted apart because the reason for our alliance had ended. We're not going to stay friendly with the same people for our entire lives and that's fine. Knowing that can also be a healthy way to view certain friendships when we think they may need to end.

One last thing, and this is really important. When evaluating a friendship, I have learned to do what I call a "Container Check." I once had someone in my life who had all good intentions of being there when I needed her. I was going through a difficult time emotionally and she would pay me great lip service about how she would always be there for me no matter what and she was completely on board with helping me through this hard time. Well, despite those well-meaning words, time and time again she was unable to be the friend for me that I needed at that time. When I was crying about this to an older and wiser person, this sage said to me, "Her container isn't big enough for you."

It was true. Her personal emotional container could only hold a certain amount, and more often than not it had no room for me. I loved that imagery because it makes the concept so tangibly clear. I still use it to this day, picturing someone with their own Tupperware-type container, filled with their stuff, and discerning whether or not there is sufficient room for others' stuff in it.

Of course the size and shape of people's containers can change depending on what's going on in their own lives—parents' containers grow exponentially when another child is born and our own containers can shrink drastically when we've experienced a devastating loss. But trying to assess the amount of extra room in someone's container can be an excellent way of determining whether or not a person could potentially disappoint you or possibly be able to buoy you in the way that you need.

So when you're choosing happiness in your life, I would encourage you to examine your relationships. If there are some that aren't interested in taking your happiness journey with you, then it may be time to decide where they need to be, or not be, on your road to joy.

Take Your Inner Child
for a Walk

And be sure to jump in some puddles along the way.

I recently took a workshop led by the great innovator Scott F. Mason* titled "Pure Imagination." In it we explored the concept of childlike fun and what that looked like to us. We realized that most childhood entertainment involved using and stretching our imagination, coupled with unabashed creativity free of worrying about what someone else will think of it.

This is why kids can play for hours with sticks and dirt and rocks in the backyard. Or why they can get together and say things like, "You're the cowboy, I'm the princess, let's play!" There's no preparation beforehand, they just jump in and enjoy themselves.

Have you ever seen a young child at a playground dashing gleefully from the swings to the slide to the monkey bars and back to the slide? It can be so inspiring to watch kids as they run and jump and enjoy themselves with enthusiastic abandon, not holding anything back because of what they think they might look like or how someone else might be judging them.

*Scott is the founder and CEO of F-ervescent Productions. www.f-ervescent .com.

They just play.

I believe that we can create pockets of happiness by injecting more play time into our adult lives. We fill our hours with work and responsibilities and social media, which leaves very little extra time for anything else; which means it's all the more important that we take the opportunities to play and have fun when we get them, and even feel free to schedule them regularly to help keep our wonderment and joy alive.

I read a story about a woman who was completely burnt out from work and stress, and as she was taking a walk during her lunch break one day, she passed a park with a swing set. She remembered how much she loved swinging on the swings as a kid, so before she could talk herself out of it, she went over, kicked off her heels, situated herself in her pencil skirt on the narrow swing, and took off.

Immediately she was back in time, as a carefree eight-year-old, pushing herself higher with every swing. She pumped her legs and threw her head back, fully immersed in the freedom and pleasure of feeling her hair blow back in the wind and her heart soaring to the sky. When she stopped after a few minutes, she said she felt refreshed and filled with happiness, along with a sense of calm and clarity that she had not felt in a very long time. I'm not sure what happened to her after that, but I remember that scene of her swinging so vividly in my mind and I return to that image often when I think about what it means to "play" as an adult.

So often playing as a grown-up involves competition, and who needs that? Why can't we get together to play cards or a board game and state right off the bat, "This is just for fun, we don't need to keep score because it doesn't matter who wins."

Why are things done "just for fun" often labeled as foolish or unworthy?

In the workshop Scott referenced an article by David Branchflower, an economist at Dartmouth, called "The U-Curve of Happiness." The research shows that:

- Happiness in youth is high.
- Reaching a peak in the twenties.
- Declines in middle age.
- Then there's an upswing again after age fifty.

There are some obvious reasons for this data. Most of us in our twenties do not have major responsibilities like raising children, paying a mortgage, or taking care of aging parents. Many of those things hit in our thirties and forties, along with more job stress as we move up in our careers. Oftentimes after we hit the half-century mark, we become empty nesters, we begin pondering retirement, and we are hopefully more comfortable financially after working for a few decades.

So, during those times when our happiness seems to naturally decline, is there a way we can combat what the research shows?

I feel very strongly that one of the best ways is to return to those activities that made us happy as children and make time to incorporate them into our daily lives as much as possible. Then, and most importantly, **not judge ourselves or care what anyone else thinks about it.**

Here are some examples of things we can do to foster our imaginations like we did when we were kids:

Play with Play-Doh. The smell alone will bring you right back to preschool.

Play with LEGOs. (Just make sure to pick any stray ones up off the floor when you're done. Stepping with bare feet on a sharp-edged plastic brick is unbelievably painful.)

Blow bubbles. This always puts me in a good mood, and I always make sure to have a bottle with the little wand in it under my kitchen sink to create some random moments of bubble magic.

The next time it rains, put on a raincoat and puddle boots and take a walk, making sure to splash in every puddle you come across.

If you live somewhere where winters come with snow, put on your snow boots and parka and go out and play! Catch snowflakes on your tongue, make snow angels, and make a snowman! (The shoveling can wait.)

Skip rocks on a pond or a lake.

Find a rock you like, bring it home, and paint it in a decorative way. Then put it somewhere in your yard or garden where you can see it often. Even better, paint several and place them around your neighborhood as impromptu art.

If you're at the beach, collect seashells and let your toes be tickled by the ocean, even if it's freezing cold. Make something like a picture frame or a sculpture with the shells you collected and display it proudly.

Can you see how important it is to do things outside in the fresh air and sunshine? Even just making sure to go outside once a day can have a wonderful effect on your mind and body.

Bake something simple, like five-ingredient cookies, and make them as big or as small as you want, without worrying about uniformity or what they look like. Then enjoy eating them, warm, with a glass of cold milk.

Make a necklace out of dried pasta and string or a macaroni art piece. Spray it with gold spray paint to make it look extra lovely.

When you're out for a walk, pay less attention to your pace and your mileage, and instead call it a "Nature Walk." Use as many of your senses as you can as you go leisurely along. Pick a dandelion, blow the seeds, and then watch them scatter until they are all gone. Watch a caterpillar creep along the sidewalk. If you pass a rose bush or a honeysuckle shrub take a moment to breathe in the sweet scents. Listen to birds chirping or water trickling and whatever other cool nature sounds you can hear. Find a leaf and carefully examine the pattern of veins on both sides. Collect a bunch of leaves, bring them home, and do a crayon rubbing on them.

Speaking of crayons, color in a coloring book or draw something with crayons, markers, or colored pencils. Then:

HANG YOUR MASTERPIECE ON THE REFRIGERATOR! Thank you, Scott, for this fantastic suggestion. Hopefully when you were young and brought home a drawing or an art project, it was proudly displayed on the refrigerator for all to see. Do the same thing with whatever you create during your play time, no matter what it looks like or no matter how "bad" you think it is. Who cares? YOU made it, so therefore it is worthy of being put on exhibition. You don't have to leave it up forever but put it up for a bit so you can be proud of what you created, and as a reminder of how much fun tapping into your childhood imagination can be.

When you're choosing happiness, choose to play like when you were a child and take time to let go of how you are "supposed" to act when you're an adult. Revisit those days of unadulterated joy when our only limit was our imagination.

Cultivate   Hope

Honor your   Aspirations

Opt for   Peace

Own your   Power

Shine with   Your

Exuberance   !!!

Channel Beyonce

For those days when you might be feeling a bit down or discouraged, I have a tried-and-true piece of advice that works every time. It is:

Channel Beyonce.

Or Dwayne "The Rock" Johnson. Or JLo. Or LeBron James. Or Clark Gable. Or whoever embodies confidence, self-assurance, and superstardom for you. Pick one of those people and invite them into your body for a bit. While they're there, take a few moments to envision what it might feel like to actually live in their shoes. If you really get into this exercise, I can tell you from experience that you will most likely feel a lift in your demeanor and an elevated way of carrying yourself. Just this small shift in feeling "who you are walking around as" can make a huge difference, even for a short time.

It really works! Now this is not to say that any of these famous people are "better" than we are. They are just people like all of us. But if we can harness the bits of them that exude power and self-confidence, we can personify those traits within ourselves. For example:

The first time I tried this I was about to run a bunch of errands and felt very low-energy and really blah all around. I didn't like that feeling, so I wondered if there was something I could do to shake myself out of my malaise and bring myself up to how I wanted to feel instead. So I thought to myself, "How would Beyonce run these errands?" (Which I realize is a silly thing to think because I doubt Beyonce runs her own errands. I'm pretty sure she has people to do those for her. But nevertheless …)

With Queen Bey in mind, I reached into my closet for a sparkly top and black pants, replacing the hoodie and workout bottoms I had been sporting thus far in my day. I took out the ponytail, put on some lip gloss, and headed out, keeping her presence squarely in the front of my brain.

When I got out of the car at stop number one, I said to myself, "I'm Beyonce. I'm Beyonce," and I felt my head pull up a little higher on my shoulders. Every step I took toward the store felt confident and assured and powerful. I involuntarily smiled as the double doors automatically opened, and I boldly stepped inside, as if they had parted just for me.

As I consciously kept this persona going, the strangest thing happened. Upon encountering a complete stranger in an aisle, he nodded at me and smiled as we passed each other. A few minutes later, another complete stranger went by and she smiled and said, "Cute top!" A short while after that, another person I did not know smiled at me and enthusiastically said, "Hi!" as if we were friends.

It was bewildering each time, but as I sat in my car afterwards to ponder my experiment, I realized that because I was putting forth an aura of confidence and joy, people around me responded to that. Had I been sending out signals of ennui or indifference, I'm sure people would have avoided me, or I would have just blended into the store surroundings.

I'm not saying that I did this to elicit a response from others—that result never even occurred to me. But seeing how my presence as a Beyonce conduit made an inspiring impact

on others drove home the point that the way we carry ourselves and the thoughts we have about it can actually make a
significant difference in our outlook, even while we're doing
mundane things.

So for those times when you just can't seem to muster up
the energy to smile or feel some measure of happiness, I would
suggest that you "fake it 'til you make it," and channel a person
who commands attention with their presence and freely dis-
plays their confidence and power to the world. Not only will it
help, but it's also a ton of fun to walk in their shoes for a while.
Hopefully, they will end up feeling so comfortable they'll be
your own shoes too.

Keep a Healthy Relationship with Social Media

First of all, let me say that I am not completely anti–social media. Social media has been a great way for me to do things like promote my music, reconnect with long-lost friends, and it has been an integral part of getting my Choose Happiness content out to people. So while I am not wholly against it, I believe it needs to be used wisely, safely, and in a way that makes it add value to people's lives, instead of becoming their reason for living.

I know someone who posts every single day, often several times per day. Her life seems to be ruled by her posts, and it seems like nothing she does "counts" until it is posted, and she gets the affirmation she's craving from other people's virtual thumbs-ups and emoji hearts. She posts when she bakes something, she posts when she's working out, she posts when the dog is sleeping on her lap, and I'm sure she posts plenty of other things that I don't know about since I stopped following her a few years ago.

I've actually stopped following a lot of people and concurrently have consciously limited my exposure to most social media due to the recent political unrest and the damaging vitriol that people feel the need to spew out into the world on a regular basis. Plus I have taken heed of the hundreds of scientific studies that have shown that human beings are happier overall when they limit their attention to social media and pay more attention to nature, a tactile hobby, and fostering connections with real, in-the-flesh humans rather than the virtual ones online.

(And I won't even get into all of the horrible scams and targeted phishing and false identity crimes that go on daily, which are out there for the express purpose to hurt and take advantage of people. Social media can be very dangerous and needs to be handled accordingly.)

But back to my former friend, who was a big catalyst in my decision to limit my social media attention. When I first met her, she would constantly complain about her husband and their terrible, toxic marriage. She would go on and on about the things they said to each other and how much she wanted to leave him. I was always the supportive friend, listening over and over and encouraging her to do what was right for her and her son.

Imagine my surprise when shortly after one of these conversations, she posted a photo of herself and her husband, smiling broadly while clinking wine glasses with the caption, "Date night with my love." Or the day after she was crying to me about something hurtful he had said, she shared a selfie of the two of them, heads together and grinning with the caption, "Me and my cute hubby. How lucky am I?"

Ugh.

She also confided in me about her son's drug use and how he had run away from home twice, and then a few months later when the holidays rolled around, there were the three of them in their blemish-free, wrinkle-free, not-a-hair-out-of-place-thanks-to-Photoshop Christmas card, hands entwined with the message, "Holiday Wishes from Our Love-Filled House to Yours."

Now clearly this woman had a pathological need to show the world that everything was spectacular in her life, regardless of what was really going on, and obviously felt the overwhelming need to create a fantasy for the outside world to see. Which has a lot to say about her own obsessive need for approval and her compulsive need to always put on a bright face for others even when it was a total lie. Which got me thinking...

Hearing one thing come out of her mouth and seeing something completely different online made me think to myself ... which one was the lie? I mean, I thought all of the negative stuff she was talking about was the truth and the photos were the lie, but what if she just wanted attention and sympathy from me and things were not actually as bad at home as she was purporting in our conversations? I'll never know and it doesn't matter, but the point is, so much of what we see on social media IS in fact a lie, and we're foolish to believe that people are posting anything other than neatly curated "highlight reels" of their lives containing only the parts that they want us to see.

I think it's really sad that so many people, especially kids, have their happiness determined by how many positive responses they get to their posts. It is also incredibly damaging and hurtful when kids are told by their friends that they aren't free to get together, and then they see those same friends posting happy selfies with other kids, sending the very clear message that certain people were deliberately left out and ostracized from a group. We're supposed to be teaching kids to live their lives authentically and genuinely, which only happens when we don't put so much stock in what other people think of us, but social media can make that nearly impossible.

Again, social media isn't inherently bad, but putting so much of our time and effort into scrolling and posting and waiting for "likes" has been proven to be unhealthy for our psyches and can be a real impediment to finding true happiness in our daily lives. Yes, it's fun to post vacation photos and inspirational quotes and to see what old friends and are up to. But when the posting and the approvals become an addiction, and we're spending more time inside on social media than outside and interacting with the world, then that's a recipe for unhappiness, and that's not what we're seeking here.

I saw this quote the other day:

Giving up social media for even just 7 days boosts happiness and reduces anger and feelings of loneliness.

I'm not suggesting giving it up entirely, unless that's what's right for you and the happiest life you can lead, but that scientific finding really puts things into perspective. Ideally we should all have enough going on in our lives and be so engrossed in our own pursuits and endeavors that we don't have time to stop and watch what other people are doing. We should be so filled up with our own happiness and contentment that we don't feel the overwhelming need to share it for others' acknowledgment or endorsement. Why should what someone else thinks of what we're doing matter so much? And why do we put so much emphasis on what we perceive other people are thinking of us? No one and nothing besides our own heart and head deserve that kind of power over our own happiness.

Here's a good test to see where you are: When you're on social media ask yourself, how does this make me feel? Am I lifted up, encouraged, joyful, excited about life, inspired, or comforted? Or does it make you feel jealous, angry, dissatisfied, anxious, downtrodden, or miserable? Really check in with yourself and make your decision based on those feelings.

Happiness is a choice, and we can always choose to put down the phone or turn off the computer. Those don't have to be guidelines in our lives because I can guarantee you, they will never bring you the true happiness you're looking for. How could they? They don't care about you, they do not have your best interests at heart, and they are not your friends, no matter how often they are by your side.

It's the Little Things that Really Do Matter

Especially the little things we do for others.

When we were living in Boston, my kids and I would frequent the restaurant Friendly's. It's a casual sit-down restaurant with an ice cream parlor attached—what could be better? The best part was, the kids' meals came with a mini sundae, so it was a favorite place for the whole family.

One day, shortly after we had been seated and my kids were industriously working on the games on the kids' menu, an older gentleman came in alone. He was seated at a small table that was tucked behind a partition that was near our table. He removed his hat, picked up his menu, then put it down and waited expectantly for someone to come and take his order.

He waited.

He waited some more.

He waited some more.

Long after our order had been taken our waitress finally saw him and said perkily, "Oops, sorry, I didn't see you there. What can I get you?"

I felt tears well up in my eyes as her offhand comment registered in my brain.

"I didn't see you there."

I could cry now just thinking about it.

It has been said that one of the most important things to all of us as human beings is to be seen and validated. To feel like the space we take up on this Planet Earth matters in some way. While this waitress's casual remark may not have upset this man at all, it definitely upset me, and I was determined to do something about it.

So a few minutes later when she arrived at our table with our food I whispered to her, "Can you please bring me that gentleman's check when he's finished eating? I'd like to pay for his meal today."

She looked at me like I had two heads.

"Um, . . . what's that?" she asked.

As quietly as I could, I repeated what I wanted, making it clear that under no circumstances was she to reveal my plan to the man, as my kids looked on, a bit confusedly.

"Ohhh," the waitress said. "But I can't bring you the check until he's finished eating and he might order ice cream."

"That's fine," I said patiently. "We'll wait; we're not in any rush."

When she left, I explained to the kids that because this man was all by himself and seemed to be lonely, we were going to pay for his lunch in the hopes that it might bring him some joy. I also wanted to make sure that it was completely anonymous, because getting thanks or credit for this deed was not something I was interested in whatsoever. (I also thought it would be much more fun this way.)

"Cool," my young son said, and resumed eating his lunch.

The gentleman did indeed enjoy some ice cream after his meal, and then when it was time for his check, I saw the waitress explaining that it was already taken care of. With her back to me I couldn't hear what she said, but I was able to see the man's reaction.

First, it was complete befuddlement. Next, it was a bit of a furrowed brow as I think she repeated that his check had been paid for by someone in the restaurant and she wished him a good rest of his day.

What happened next, I can still see in my mind's eye like it happened yesterday. A smile slowly spread across his face and a light shone from his eyes. He picked up his hat, and as he put it on his head he stood up and looked carefully around the entire restaurant. At this point I made sure to be looking very intently at the word find on the kids' menu in front of me and putting the crayons back into their tiny box. When I looked up again, he was walking slowly toward the exit, continuing to crane his head around and smiling from ear to ear. He was still smiling as he pushed the door open to leave, and I could see that he was standing slightly taller than when he had entered and had the tiniest bit of a spring in his step as he went to his car.

I held back the tears as the waitress approached with both of our checks.

"Wow!" she said, "You really made that guy's day."

I smiled and said, "Thanks so much for your help; we couldn't have done it without you."

She smiled brightly back and went off with a little bounce in her step as well.

I looked at the man's bill. It was $9.61.

$9.61 to bring someone some unexpected joy.

$9.61 to make sure someone knew that they were seen.

$9.61 to send someone the message that they mattered.

$9.61, which lifted up yet another person, the waitress, who was now happier because she had helped to make a joyful difference in someone else's life.

And most importantly, $9.61 to show my kids how powerful it can be to take the time and effort to show someone else, even a complete stranger, some love and consideration.

That's $9.61 well spent, if you ask me.

Which brings me to the concept of . . .

The Blessing Fund

That experiment at Friendly's spearheaded a practice in our family that we call The Blessing Fund.

Every year we set aside a portion of money—some years it's been a little, some years it's been more—specifically to bless other people. Here are the rules around it:

1. It has to be something unique and different besides just giving it to a charity (which we also do, just not under this heading).
2. It has to be something tangible that will hopefully make a positive difference in someone's life.
3. It cannot be used on anything for ourselves.
4. It has to be anonymous.
5. We have to use it all up by the end of the year.

Having these parameters is really helpful, because it keeps us on the lookout for blessing opportunities throughout the year. It also helps us to consciously spend it, because we've mandated that we have to.

Why am I including this in a book about choosing happiness? It is not to show how altruistic we are or to garner admiration from you the reader. Not at all. This is why the blessings have to be anonymous; we're not interested in kudos or commendation. The reason why I'm mentioning this is because we have found that these acts of kindness bring us mountainous amounts of joy, and it's even brought us to sheer giddiness at times, especially during the holidays.

Here are some examples of The Blessing Fund in action:

After the horrific movie theater shooting in Aurora, CO, we purchased a bunch of movie tickets, gathered up some friends, and stood outside of movie theaters, handing them out to people as they walked by. This was my husband's idea. He called it "Take Back the Movies" with the intention of spreading some light after what had happened so dreadfully in the dark.

Every year on September 11th, my husband will use some of the Blessing Fund to get a gift card at a coffee shop and instruct the cashier to pay for as many customers as possible with the amount purchased. Sometimes he'll go to several coffee shops on that day, again with the purpose of infusing some joy into a difficult day.

I happen to love school supplies, and I get immense joy from combing through the back-to-school aisles to fill backpacks for local supply drives.

During the holiday season, we delight in taking gift requests from "Giving Trees" at schools or malls, and we always bring our kids to help purchase and wrap holiday presents for those families in need. **It's vitally important to include our kids in these practices and teach them that it's our responsibility to help take care of our fellow humans.** They look forward to the Giving Tree excursion every year, and it's great to see their excitement as they try to find the perfect gifts for kids they will never even meet.

We still pick up the tab for someone's meal if they are eating alone and look like they could use a lift to their spirits.

Seeing the unexpected elation on their face and watching them walk out with their head held higher on their shoulders never gets old, and it continues to fill me with as much joy as they feel, or possibly even more.

Our local ice cream place called Sweet Cow* has a great practice where every employee has a certain quota of free ice cream cones that they have to give away during their shift. On two occasions I have been the recipient of their kindness, and even such a little thing has made me feel incredibly happy and special. (The ice cream tastes better too!) So, I know firsthand just how much this kind of thing can mean to someone, and I love getting the chance to give someone else that gift of feeling honored and appreciated, just because they're alive.

For some guaranteed joy, I would suggest giving someone else a boost by doing something tangible to make a happy difference in their day. Pay for the person behind you in the drive thru. Drop off some new toys at a day care center and see the kids' reactions. Contribute to someone's crowdfunding campaign for a business they want to start. It doesn't have to have a huge price tag, but the happiness you will feel is truly priceless.

*www.sweetcowicecream.com

Laughter Is Indeed the Best Medicine

The following is an excerpt from an article by Lawrence Robinson, Melinda Smith, and Jeanne Segal.* It really encapsulates the importance of laughter in our lives from a scientific point of view, which can be helpful when looking at why it's so vital to a happy existence.

Laughter Is the Best Medicine

It's fun to share a good laugh, but did you know it can actually improve your health? Learn how to harness the powerful benefits of laughter and humor.

It's true: laughter is strong medicine. It draws people together in ways that trigger healthy physical and emotional changes in the body. Laughter strengthens your immune system, boosts mood, diminishes pain, and protects you from the damaging effects of stress. Nothing works faster or more dependably to bring your mind and body back into balance than a good laugh. Humor

---

*"Laughter Is the Best Medicine," Lawrence Robinson, Melinda Smith, M.A., and Jeanne Segal, Ph.D., HelpGuide, https://www.helpguide.org /articles/mental-health/laughter-is-the-best-medicine.htm. Updated October 2020.

lightens your burdens, inspires hope, connects you to others, and keeps you grounded, focused, and alert. It also helps you release anger and forgive sooner. . . .

The ability to laugh easily and frequently is a tremendous resource for surmounting problems, enhancing your relationships, and supporting both physical and emotional health. Best of all, this priceless medicine is fun, free, and easy to use.

As children, we used to laugh hundreds of times a day, but as adults, life tends to be more serious and laughter more infrequent. But by seeking out more opportunities for humor and laughter, you can improve your emotional health, strengthen your relationships, find greater happiness—and even add years to your life.

Laughter Is Good for Your Physical Health
Laughter relaxes the whole body. A good, hearty laugh relieves physical tension and stress, leaving your muscles relaxed for up to 45 minutes after.

Laughter boosts the immune system. Laughter decreases stress hormones and increases immune cells and infection-fighting antibodies, thus improving your resistance to disease.

Laughter triggers the release of endorphins, the body's natural feel-good chemicals. Endorphins promote an overall sense of well-being and can even temporarily relieve pain.

Laughter protects the heart. Laughter improves the function of blood vessels and increases blood flow, which can help protect you against a heart attack and other cardiovascular problems.

Laughter burns calories. . . . It's no replacement for going to the gym, but one study found that laughing for 10 to 15 minutes a day can burn approximately 40 calories—which could be enough to lose three or four pounds over the course of a year.

Laughter lightens anger's heavy load. Nothing diffuses anger and conflict faster than a shared laugh. Looking at the funny side can put problems into perspective and enable you to move on from confrontations without holding onto bitterness or resentment.

Laughter may even help you to live longer. A study in Norway found that people with a strong sense of humor outlived those who don't laugh as much. The difference was particularly notable for those battling cancer.

Laughter Helps You Stay Mentally Healthy

Laughter makes you feel good. And this positive feeling remains with you even after the laughter subsides. Humor helps you keep a positive, optimistic outlook through difficult situations, disappointments, and loss.

More than just a respite from sadness and pain, laughter gives you the courage and strength to find new sources of meaning and hope. Even in the most difficult of times, a laugh—or even simply a smile—can go a long way toward making you feel better. . . .

The Link Between Laughter and Mental Health

Laughter stops distressing emotions. You can't feel anxious, angry, or sad when you're laughing.

Laughter helps you relax and recharge. It reduces stress and increases energy, enabling you to stay focused and accomplish more.

Laughter shifts perspective, allowing you to see situations in a more realistic, less threatening light. A humorous perspective creates psychological distance, which can help you avoid feeling overwhelmed and diffuse conflict.

Laughter draws you closer to others, which can have a profound effect on all aspects of your mental and emotional health.

Laughter Brings People Together and Strengthens Relationships

There's a good reason why TV sitcoms use laugh tracks: laughter is contagious. You're . . . more likely to laugh around other people than when you're alone. And the more laughter you bring into your own life, the happier you and those around you will feel. . . .

Most laughter doesn't come from hearing jokes, but rather simply from spending time with friends and family. And it's this social aspect that plays such an important role in the health benefits of laughter. You can't enjoy a laugh with other people unless you take the time to really engage with them. When you care about someone enough to switch off your phone and really connect face to face, you're engaging in a process that rebalances the nervous system and puts the brakes on defensive stress responses like "fight or flight." And if you share a laugh as well, you'll both feel happier, more positive, and more relaxed—even if you're unable to alter a stressful situation.

How Laughing Together Can Strengthen Relationships

Shared laughter is one of the most effective tools for keeping relationships fresh and exciting. All emotional sharing builds strong and lasting relationship bonds, but sharing laughter also adds joy, vitality, and resilience. And humor is a powerful and effective way to heal resentments, disagreements, and hurts. Laughter unites people during difficult times.

Humor and playful communication strengthen our relationships by triggering positive feelings and fostering emotional connection. . . . Humor and laughter in relationships allows you to:

Be more spontaneous. . . .
Let go of defensiveness. . . .
Release inhibitions. . . .
Express your true feelings. . . .

How to Bring More Laughter into Your Life

Laughter is your birthright, a natural part of life that is innate and inborn. Infants begin smiling during the first weeks of life and laugh out loud within months of being born. Even if you did not grow up in a household where laughter was a common sound, you can learn to laugh at any stage of life.

Begin by setting aside special times to seek out humor and laughter, as you might with exercising, and build from there. Eventually, you'll want to incorporate humor and laughter into the fabric of your life, finding it naturally in everything.

Here are some ways to start:

Smile. Smiling is the beginning of laughter, and like laughter, it's contagious. When you look at someone or see something even mildly pleasing, practice smiling.

Instead of looking down at your phone, look up and smile at people. ... Notice the effect on others.

Count your blessings. Literally make a list. The simple act of considering the positive aspects of your life will distance you from negative thoughts that block humor and laughter. ...

When you hear laughter, move toward it. Sometimes humor and laughter are private, a shared joke among a small group, but usually not. More often, people are very happy to share something funny because it gives them an opportunity to laugh again and feed off the humor you find in it. When you hear laughter, seek it out and ask, "What's funny?"

Spend time with fun, playful people. These are people who laugh easily—both at themselves and at life's absurdities—and who routinely find the humor in everyday events. Their playful point of view and laughter are contagious. Even if you don't consider yourself a lighthearted, humorous person, you can still seek out people who like to laugh and make others laugh. ...

Bring humor into conversations. Ask people, "What's the funniest thing that happened to you today? This week? In your life?"

Simulated Laughter

... It's possible to laugh without experiencing a funny event—and simulated laughter can be just as beneficial as the real thing. It can even make exercise more fun and productive. A Georgia State University study found that incorporating bouts of simulated laughter into an exercise program helped improve older adults' mental health as

well as their aerobic endurance. Plus, hearing others laugh
... can often trigger genuine laughter.

To add simulated laughter into your own life, search
for laugh yoga or laugh therapy groups. Or you can start
simply by laughing at other people's jokes, even if you
don't find them funny. Both you and the other person will
feel good, it will draw you closer together, and who knows,
it may even lead to some spontaneous laughter.

Creating opportunities to laugh:

- Watch a funny movie, TV show, or YouTube video
- Invite friends or co-workers out to a comedy club
- Read the funny pages
- Seek out funny people
- Share a good joke or a funny story
- Check out your bookstore's humor section
- Host game night with friends
- Play with a pet
- Goof around with children
- Do something silly
- Make time for fun activities ...

Don't go a day without laughing. Think of it like exercise or breakfast and make a conscious effort to find
something each day that makes you laugh. Set aside ten
to fifteen minutes and do something that amuses you. The
more you get used to laughing each day, the less effort
you'll have to make.

...

As laughter, humor, and play become integrated into
your life, your creativity will flourish and new opportunities

for laughing . . . will occur to you daily. Laughter takes you to a higher place where you can view the world from a more relaxed, positive, and joyful perspective.

Laughter heals, comforts, inspires, and enlivens the world around you. Make the choice to laugh as much and as often as you can.

Look at Your Resume

To remind yourself of what you are capable of.

Ordinarily I am a big proponent of the saying, "Don't look back, you're not going that way." Nine times out of ten I think it is vitally important to leave the past behind us and focus on the present moment, as well as the future, especially if the time we're in right now is particularly difficult. However, I do believe that sometimes looking at our past selves can actually be helpful, if we do it thoughtfully and purposefully.

When is that? It's when looking back at our accomplishments and triumphs can remind us of what we are capable of and what therefore can be possible for us again.

One way to do this is to look at your resume. A few years ago, I was interviewing for a job and I needed to update my resume. I pulled it up and instead of just jumping right in to see what was missing, I took a minute to really **examine** it. I read through my skills, the positions I've held, the goals I met … and not to toot my own horn or sound egotistical, but I was kind of impressed with what I had done over the years. I also had forgotten about some things for which I had won awards and received positive feedback about, and it was great to get a reminder of those too. So often I think we get mired down in focusing on what we haven't done yet, or the mistakes we've made along the way, so it can be extremely helpful (and fun) to see all of the good things we HAVE done, and how we used our talents and knowledge in beneficial ways throughout our careers and our lives.

A resume doesn't have to be work-related. If your work resume doesn't inspire you then compile your own personal resume, filled with the things you have done as a parent, a friend, a family member, a volunteer, as an athlete or an artist—you can put *anything* on there that makes you feel good about yourself and showcases your achievements. Then stand back and take a good long look at it and realize that the person who did all of those things already can certainly create and manifest any dream or goal that she or he chooses. The proof is right there in front of you.

So, while I don't believe it's healthy spend a lot of time looking back wistfully, every now and then it can be inspiring to remind ourselves of what we've achieved, what we've conquered, and what stumbling blocks we turned into stepping-stones. We can then turn our focus forward, strengthened by what we've already done, to the next awesome thing we can add to our resume.

Honor Your Free Time

Spend your free time the way you like,
not the way you think you're supposed to.
—Susan Cain

Or, more simply put, DON'T SHOULD ALL OVER YOURSELF.

This can be hard. It sits squarely in the same camp as comparison, robbing us of our own joy. But we are bombarded every day by what we "should" be doing with our time, as if invisible judgers were following us around constantly making negative comments about our choices and activities.

Who needs that?

Here's an example: I remember a conversation I had with a mom of two young kids. We were out having coffee, and at one point she leaned over the table and whispered to me, "I know this is really bad, but Charlie hasn't been sleeping and after I dropped the him off at preschool school yesterday I came home, got into bed, and watched three episodes of *Grey's Anatomy* before I had to go pick him up." I was like, "That's great! Did you feel better afterwards?" She replied shamefacedly, "Well yeah, but I should have gone to the gym, I should have started the laundry, I should have done the breakfast dishes, I should have done my emails . . . but all I did was sit and watch TV!" She felt so guilty and terrible about taking that restful and rejuvenating time for herself because she felt like she should have been doing something else.

But maybe that's why "free" time is called that. Because we're FREE (translate to ALLOWED) to spend it any way that we like. Period. It's nobody else's business what you like to do in your free time and it's not your business what someone else likes to do during theirs.

Why is this so hard? Why do we set impossible standards for ourselves in which we don't allow ourselves time to really do what we enjoy? In order to really choose happiness for ourselves we need to turn off those voices in our heads that tell us that what we like to do with our free time isn't enough. We need to banish those mental naysayers who try to make us feel inadequate or incompetent, especially when all we're trying to do is what we feel is best for us at a given time. We only get so much free time in a week or a month or a year—when it's yours, spend it doing what makes YOU happy. The dishes and the laundry will still be there, I promise.

The Power of Nicknames

Here's a great tip for dealing with difficult people in our lives. Give them a nickname.

It really works! Oftentimes we don't have a choice about keeping challenging people in our lives. In these cases, we have to make the choice about how we deal with them, while keeping ourselves as unaffected and sane as possible. I have found that giving these undesirable people funny, silly, or appropriate nicknames makes a huge difference in how I feel about our necessary interactions. It doesn't change them one bit, but it certainly helps me and my outlook on my life.

Here's an example: For four years straight I had to deal with an extremely cruel, insensitive, and disrespectful woman who was the head parent for my daughter's high school marching band. As an active parent volunteer, I had to interact with this woman on a regular basis. After several exchanges that left me either in tears or emphatically seething, I thought of one of the meanest characters I could think of and assigned her this nickname:

Nellie Oleson. From the *Little House* books by Laura Ingalls Wilder. Nellie was mean, vindictive, and rude, and this woman embodied all of those sinister traits. Interestingly, as soon as I bestowed that nickname on her, things changed. Not for her, but for ME.

I'd see her name in my inbox and when I clicked on it I could say to myself, "What does Nellie want now?" and kind of chuckle to myself. At an event where I was sitting with another mom volunteer, at one point she leaned over to me and whispered, "Uh oh, Nellie at one o'clock," and I was able to giggle for a moment, instead of instantly getting upset and stressed at the thought of her entering the room. Honestly, it made all the difference in the world when it came to dealing with this person because even though I couldn't change the situation and I certainly couldn't change her, *I could change the way I thought about it and dealt with it.*

Another example: Years ago I worked with a woman who was miserable and unkind and gave off an aura of unpleasantness wherever she went. People would turn the other way when they saw her coming down the hall, and collective eyes rolled whenever she arrived for a meeting. Unfortunately, I had to deal with her fairly frequently so she got the moniker "The Troll." I'm not sure why, it just seemed to fit. Then when she was grumbling down the hallway or doing her best to blame other people for her mistakes I could say to myself, "There goes The Troll!" Or, "The Troll is at it again!" and that allowed me to make light of the situation and not let it bother me. Again, she wasn't changing, but I was doing what I could for myself to make the best of a difficult situation.

So, I would encourage you, for those people in our lives who make it their goal to sabotage our happiness at every turn, give them a nickname. It can make the Nellies and The Trolls in our world a little bit easier to bear.

Happiness is a choice—not a result.
Nothing will make you happy until you
choose to be happy. No person will make
you happy unless you decide to be happy.
Your happiness will not come to you.
It can only come from you.

—RALPH MARSTON

Savor the Joy

This is self-explanatory but something vital to think about and remember as we go along the routines of our days:

> *Savor the joy*
> *The time it goes so fast,*
> *Savor the joy*
> *Make every moment last.*

These are lyrics from a song I wrote a few years ago for my holiday album. It describes deliberately stopping ourselves in the midst of the hustle and bustle of the holiday season and consciously focusing on enjoying the true moments of happiness among all of the trappings.

This concept can also apply to everyday life. We are so caught up in our daily duties—rushing from work to taking the kids to soccer practice to cooking dinner to helping with homework to answering emails to taking care of our parents, etc., etc., etc. Some of us have schedules that are so filled with To-Dos that we can't remember the last time we savored anything.

Most of the things on our list are non-negotiable, so while we're doing them I hope we can savor the bits of joy that come along with our ever-increasingly busy agendas.

How can we do this? By consciously stopping to be mindful during those hectic and demanding times.

When I used to drive my kids to school in the mornings, sometimes at red lights I'd put down the windows and say, "Hey guys—can you hear the birds chirping in the trees?" Then as we sat there for thirty seconds or so, we got to connect with nature, listening to the cheerful (or contentious, we never really knew) sounds of birds we couldn't even see. My daughter makes "one second a day" video diaries, which causes her to stop at some point during her day to record something of interest to then look back on at the year's end. When I am out to dinner with friends and we're all laughing uproariously at something, I always make sure to stop and look around at everyone to mentally capture that split second of collective joy.

Life is made up of precious moments that add up to an intentionally happy life. Take the time to savor those moments as often as you can.

Dance It Out

Man was I upset today. And yesterday. And the day before. I'm in a situation where I am being continually frustrated and disappointed by people that I am depending on to help me, and for a variety of reasons things aren't going as expected. This is on the heels of a thing a few days ago where there were other difficult and discouraging things going on. My mind and spirit have been taking a beating and today felt like the last straw.

There I was, crying, balling my hands into fists, and seriously considering banging my head against the nearest wall, when one of my favorite songs, "Shut Up and Dance" by Walk the Moon, came on the radio.

The words from Shonda Rhimes and *Grey's Anatomy* came into my head: Dance it out!

I turned up the volume, moved away from the open windows, and proceeded to have an energetic, high-spirited, completely all-out three-minute dance party with myself.

I whirled my arms, I moved my hips, I spun around, and even jumped up and down to the beat of the song. I danced and danced for all I was worth, and when the song was over, I caught my breath and noticed how I was feeling.

Light and sparkly from head to toe.

My problems were still there, I still had a difficult email to send, the fact that my trust had been broken multiple times still existed, but I felt so much better about it all. I was calmer, and therefore able to deal with the situation more rationally, I had some adrenaline flowing, which gave me a more positive outlook on things, and the feeling of my heart pumping and my limbs and body moving made me feel powerful and alive and like I could handle any difficulty that came my way . . . at least for the next hour or so.

I learned some very important things from this little exercise:

1. When you're facing a difficult situation, allow yourself to take a break from it and gain some perspective. Watch a show or video that makes you laugh, listen to music that you like, go for a walk, bake some brownies, clean out a closet, do SOMETHING that will take you out of the situation and that will keep you from sinking down deeper into the hole you're halfway down into already. Removing yourself from it and focusing your eyes and your brain on something else, even for a few minutes, will help you to get a different outlook and hopefully even help get your brain in the right mode to find a solution.

2. Do something physical! Be active! When James Taylor talked about overcoming his drug addiction, he said that what he found to be most effective was to "sweat it out." Find an activity you enjoy doing and sweat out the anxiety and the stress and the feeling like you don't have control over your current situation. This isn't "go work out to improve your looks." It's do something that will remind you that you have a body that works and that you're a strong, capable person. It will also give you an energy boost to help you conquer the problem that's facing you at the moment.

3. Dancing in particular can be very therapeutic. The act of moving your body to music invigorates the senses and allows

a very specific instance of "letting go" to occur. You can also let go in this way through meditation or yoga or a spin class, but dancing—when you are allowing your body to move freely, the way it wants to, with no prescribed routine—is very freeing for the mind, body, and soul. There's something about moving one's corporal self through space and time that connects us to the Earth and the atmosphere around us, and it can be a very spiritual experience that allows for an opening of our hearts to possibilities previously unseen.

No matter how hard we try to control the world around us, bad things are going to happen. Things aren't going to go according to plan, people will disappoint us, and even though we try not to, we will sometimes take things personally and be hurt by them. How we deal with these things is vitally important to our mental well-being—we can curl up in a ball and bemoan the state of our lives, or we can dance it out and figure out the next step to solve the problem at hand. Sometimes we forget we have that choice, but we always do.

Today I am making the choice to dance it out! Care to join me?

Experience Art — Live!

I just finished watching the Pavarotti documentary by Ron Howard and not only was it an incredible film, but I found myself bawling—BAWLING—at the very end, when Pavarotti's famous rendition of "Nessun Dorma" is shown in its entirety. I had teared up near the end when his death was described, but even the sadness of that did not bring me to sobbing, as this moment did, causing the dog to turn to look at me as if to say, "Is everything okay? Do I need to call someone?"

Many years ago I had the incredible opportunity to see the Maestro sing live (I actually got to meet him briefly afterwards, but that is a story for another day) and it was one of those exceptionally special times in my life where I felt transported to another plane just from being in that space and hearing his magnificent voice soar into the rafters and envelop all of us. These kinds of live cultural experiences can significantly lift our spirits and cause a positive change in our outlook on life, sometimes with lifelong lasting effects.

I can remember seeing the original cast perform *Les Miserable*s on Broadway. (Shout out to say a huge THANK YOU to my parents for that transformative experience!) Toward the end of the show when Valjean sang "Bring Him Home," on the very last note I found my teenaged self with real tears in my eyes. Yes, everyone had been killed and it's a devastating moment plot-wise, but it wasn't that. It was the music and the exquisite, unmatchable beauty of Colm Wilkinson's ethereal high note at the end that caused a seismic shift within my body and generated a visceral emotional reaction. That was the first time I realized the immense power of experiencing something artistic live, and how it can truly touch a person's very soul.

I always feel greatly inspired after seeing a very good production of a musical or a play or a concert. The exhilaration of it all leaves me feeling like I've been spending time on a different, higher level somehow, and it's because of the shared, in-person experience that cannot be easily described and can never be replicated.

Question: Why is it that bands and solo artists always sound so much better on recordings than they do live, and yet we still love to see them in concert?

Because it's the collective experience of BEING THERE, hearing the music, dancing around, and enjoying yourself **with other people** (more on this in the chapter on Collective Joy) that sparks inspiration within us. It's also the miraculous knowledge that we are all sharing this one special moment in time and space that will never be repeated. Even if the set list is the same the next night and the next night and the one after that, the show will be different based on the feeling from the crowd, the emotions of the performers, the weather outside, what's going on in the world, etc. To experience a live, never-to-be-seen-nor-felt-the-same-way-again event is extremely powerful. Which is why I would encourage you to take in those experiences as often as you can.

Have you noticed that when you try to show your friends the videos you took at a concert, they don't translate the thrill and excitement you felt while you were there? That's because you can't capture an immersive, 360-degree, full sensory experience on a tiny flat screen with miniscule speakers. It's impossible to communicate what it's like being a part of something so big and exhilarating and special. As human beings I believe we are designed to relish the bliss that comes with these exceptional moments of shared abundant joy with complete strangers, who become our partners in living life for a brief time.

Well-intentioned and superbly executed art can truly be magical. Whether it's a show on a stage, a musical concert, a cinematic film, a fine arts exhibit in a museum, a photography show, or a weaving or quilt exhibition in a barn, art is meant to inspire us. It's designed to evoke emotions and light the fires within us that can lie dormant when our attention is taken up solely by what's showing up on our social media feeds. It can shift our eyes and ears from the inundation of political buzzwords and celebrity drivel, to the beauty of what's possible for us and for our fellow humans.

If we're choosing happiness in our lives then we are also choosing to make a conscious effort to fill our lives with things that fill up our senses, that tap into our emotions, and that keep us on a path of constantly seeking the good out in the world. So, make the choice to buy those concert tickets for the musician that you love. Make the choice to make a trip to your nearby city to see the touring company of the Broadway show you really want to see. Take a day off from work and spend it at a museum, drinking in the miracles you see when mere mortals take a blank piece of canvas or a shapeless piece of clay and transform it into something brilliant and awe-inspiring. Open yourself up to the art around you, and even if it's not something that you particularly like, you will still have the experience of doing it and being exposed to it.

The best part of experiencing art in person is that it can inspire you to create something artistic yourself. To take that pottery or drawing class you've always wanted to take so you can express yourself in that way. To audition for the community theater that's putting on a play. To explore your surroundings with your camera and experiment with different filters and lighting. Or whatever sparks interest in you artistically.

To quote Luciano Pavarotti: *"Life is too short."*

I completely agree, Maestro. And while we're here I believe we should take opportunities to experience art in as many ways we can, as collectively as we can. To truly experience it, savor it, be immersed in it, and enjoy it.

Talk to Your Elders, and Listen to Them

There is something that if you take the time to do it, it will most likely bring you happiness and give you a different perspective about your world, which we all could use from time to time. It's this:

Ask your grandparents (or great-grandparents, or great-aunts and great-uncles) questions about their youth, and then listen attentively to the answers. Even better, record their answers for future generations. It's fun, incredibly interesting, and you'll get the added benefit of brightening your relative's day, especially one who might not be included in things very often anymore.

One of the most fascinating conversations I've ever had was with my husband's ninety-five-year-old grandmother shortly before she passed away. While her body had slowed down a bit by then, her mind was still as sharp as ever. We spent an afternoon with her, asking her question after question about her very intriguing upbringing, which led to her pulling out dusty photo albums and telling us nicknames for her boarding school friends which hadn't been invoked in more than eighty years. When she passed away less than a year later, we were all so grateful that we had gotten to spend that exquisitely special time with her, getting a glimpse into her past, long before marriage, her six children, and her many grandchildren were even a glimmering speck in her consciousness.

I encourage you to seek out your older relatives or older honorary family members to find out about the lives they lived long before you knew them. Not only will you be regaled with stories that would seem next to impossible now, but you will be giving them the gift of reaching back into their memories and drawing out beloved people and experiences long forgotten. It was wonderful to see Grandma's face brighten with the mention of a dear friend from her childhood, and so much fun to see her engulfed in laughter when recalling a funny memory of a prank she and her friends pulled on an unsuspecting housemother. Everyone loves to talk about themselves, and the people we know now as slow-moving and perhaps-sometimes-old-fashioned senior citizens can really come alive when asked about the good times of their youth. Conversations like these can really put things in perspective for grandkids and great grandkids, as they can see their elders in a different light.

Here are some suggestions for questions to ask your older relatives:

- What toys did you play with as a child?
- What was your favorite place to visit as a youngster?
- What was your favorite outfit to wear as a kid?
- Did you or your siblings/friends have nicknames? What were they?
- What were your household chores?
- Did you get an allowance? If so, how much was it?
- Did your parents have any specific rules (e.g., dinner was always at a specific time, never touch the thermostat, a set curfew, etc.)?
- Did you have a beloved pet when you were young?

- What was the best birthday or holiday gift you received?
- What were some of your family traditions growing up?
- What was your favorite subject in school?
- How did you spend your free time?
- Do you remember the cost of anything that you wanted to buy (e.g., candy bars, comic books, school supplies, etc.)?
- Where did you attend school, and what was it like?
- What was your first job?
- What is the biggest innovation that you've seen in your lifetime (e.g., telephones, televisions, computers, motor cars, etc.)?

These are just a few suggestions. Feel free to come up with your own about whatever you want to know. I also encourage you to allow the conversation to go off into tangents—oftentimes the best stories come out of memories that aren't specifically tied to a particular questions. We heard plenty of hilarious anecdotes that I didn't even ask about, so it can be really fun to start with your questions and then just sit back and enjoy listening.

This is one of those things that many of us mean to do but never get around to actually doing. It's worth your time, I promise you, and you will gain knowledge and viewpoints that will broaden your mental scope and give you extraordinary things to ponder and realize about times gone by. This kind of perspective can be invaluable in our choosing happiness journey, by getting us out of our current thoughts and providing us with different views of what is possible, no matter what era a person has lived in.

Live Your Life

Allow me to explain what I mean by that.

A few years ago I was working out with a trainer, and to change things up a bit, we devised a game where we would stand in the gym a few feet apart and toss and bounce a ball back and forth to each other while standing on one foot. (This was to help with balance and core strength.) One day toward the end of a workout he asked me if there was something specific that I wanted to do and I was like, "Oooh, let's play the ball game in the gym!" So we started playing, and sometimes I would miss the ball and have to run after it, dodging other people in the space, and then I started making up silly rules and I was giggling and laughing the whole time, and at one point he stopped, held the ball in his hands, looked at me, and said, "Wow, you are really enjoying this." And I was like, "Yeah, it's so much fun!" And then he broke into a big smile and said, "This is called living life."

That same year I worked for a week at a remote camp up in the mountains. When I arrived and got the tour of the place, several people said to me, "You've got to go out to the tennis courts at night and look up at the stars. They are amazing way out there." I made a mental note of that because there are few things that I enjoy as much as looking up at the stars at night. The week went on, and when I got to the last night I realized that I had never taken the time to go out and see the stars and I really didn't want to miss out on that experience. I was a little afraid to go by myself since I only had a rough idea of where the tennis courts were, and the cell service was spotty at best. So, after dinner I went up to another teacher and asked him if he would accompany me later to go out and look at the stars. He happily agreed, admitting that he wasn't so sure exactly where the tennis courts were either.

Figuring that between the two of us we'd be able to find them, we set off after dark, almost immediately regretting our complete cluelessness with regard to bringing a flashlight. We used our phone lights to illuminate our way, scrambling through overgrown brush and nearly tumbling down a hill to find these ever-elusive tennis courts. We finally got there, giggling the entire time as we stumbled through the gate and found a place to settle down to look up at the sparkling night sky. As we propped ourselves up against our guitar cases, the guy looked over at me and said, "This is called living life."

I thought it was interesting that two people, neither of whom I knew very well, made the same exact observation using the same exact words. That got me thinking ... I wonder if I do things slightly differently than other people at times. For example, I have been known to stop my kids in their tracks in the early morning rush out the door to take a moment to witness a breathtaking sunrise. On a recent nighttime drive to South Dakota when it was pitch black on the road, we all stepped out of the car into the frigid night air to look up at the gorgeous array of stars that could be seen in our distant location. We did the same thing when we visited the Grand Canyon, getting out of the car and using our phone lights as a guide as we carefully picked our way through a nearby forest, taking care to notice bear traps along the way.

Doing these kinds of things are very regular for my family and me. It's perfectly normal for us to be in various corners of the house and then someone will yell "Sunset!" and we'll all come running to see it together. Even though my kids are older now, whenever we go to a beach, we will always construct a sandcastle together, complete with moat, and then stay long enough to watch the tide come and fill it in. We always take what we call a "Leaf Drive," in the Fall, making sure to take in the magnificence of the changing colors of the leaves on the trees—maples and oaks in the Pacific Northwest and New England, and now aspens in the Rocky Mountains.

While these things are simply a part of how we choose to live our lives, when they are pointed out to me, it makes me wonder how many of us are rushing along from one thing to another, and not taking the time to notice the beauty of nature or to see the humor in a particular situation. Not that I am saying that this is something that everyone should do or how people should live their lives—I know that this kind of pausing to take in the little things or to proverbially "smell the roses" isn't for everyone. But if you feel like you are caught up on a hamster wheel and can't quite find your way off, maybe stopping on your way home to look up at the stars after working late could be a way for you to take a moment to absorb the bigger picture and get some peaceful perspective. Or maybe if you work near a playground, take a few minutes during your lunch break to climb onto the swings and feel the wind in your hair like when you were a kid. Or it can be as simple as making the choice to take out your earbuds and forgo listening to music or a podcast on a walk so you can be fully present and embrace your natural surroundings. It may take some practice, but choosing to deliberately do these things, replacing other elements of our regular rushed routine, can make a big difference in the happiness in our lives.

Life is meant to be fun, joyous, and fulfilling.
—Jim Henson

After all, "This is called living life."

Try Something New

I love asking people this question:

What would you try if you knew you could not fail?

Really think about this. What have you always wanted to do but were afraid to try?

Figuring this out could be a key step in choosing happiness in your life.

Here are some of the answers I've received:

Start my own business.
Plant a garden.
Learn a new language.
Ice-skate.
Become a vegan.
Sing.
Build a house from the ground up.
Foster a child.
Travel someplace exotic.
Paint on a giant canvas.
Design and sew my own clothes.
Go back to school.
Write a book.
Try stand-up comedy.
Train for a marathon.
Make watches.
Juggle.

Build a ship.
Ask someone out.
Go to cooking school.
Tile a shower.
Get a dog.

Now that you've seen those ideas, maybe they are sparking some things that you have always wanted to try doing but the fear of failure has gotten in your way. To that I ask you these questions:

1. What's on your list?
2. Would attempting something on your list bring you joy?
3. Could you allow yourself to experience the joy of trying it, even though you might not be successful at it right away?

If the answer to question 2 or 3 is yes, then my only question left for you is:

What are you waiting for?

Get Out of a Rut

The more we get stuck in our usual routines, the harder it can be to try something new, but it can be so important in consciously choosing happiness for ourselves. Sometimes we forget to have fun and shake things up when our lives are so busy, so we end up needing to make an effort to embrace spontaneity.

When author and comedian Katie Goodman* teaches her improvisation workshop she talks about the extraordinary gift we can give ourselves of being spontaneous. When we make spontaneity a practice in our brains, it trains that part of the brain to bypass its own censor—also known as our inner critic—and when that is circumvented, we're able to foster innovation. Silencing that voice that tells us we're not good enough or we shouldn't try something allows creative ideas to burst through, and we feel free to go for things, even though we might not be good at them the first time around. The absence of that unwelcome opinion in our heads helps us to give up perfectionism and provides us with the freedom we need to seek the happiness we could enjoy from a new experience.

So how can we practice spontaneity? Change up the familiar. Take a different route to go someplace regular like the grocery store or the post office. It may take longer to get there

*Katie's work can be found at www.katiegoodman.com and www.katie goodmanspeaking.com.

(so don't try this when you're in a hurry), so take that extra time to notice the unfamiliar scenery around you. Actively doing something like this can be a great exercise for opening ourselves up to new experiences, and it's a low-risk way to start practicing looking at our lives with new eyes.

Play the "Turn Right, Turn Left" game in the car. The person in the passenger seat gets blindfolded and the driver starts driving. At every stop sign or traffic light, the passenger instructs the driver to turn right or turn left without looking at where they are. Play the game for whatever period of time you have designated beforehand, and then when the time is up, everyone in the car goes for lunch or dinner at the first establishment you see at the end of the route. It's a ton of fun, and it shows the exciting possibilities of what can happen when you're spontaneous and allow things to occur randomly. In this game we always find interesting places that we would have never found otherwise, and even if it's not the best meal of our lives, it's still a new and different experience to appreciate and enjoy together.

There are so many other ways to do this if you're feeling stagnant in your life. If you're bored at work, think about what you've always wanted to do and check job listings in that field. Even if you can't leave your current job right away it can be inspiring to know that there are other jobs out there that could be more satisfying to you in the future.

If you're a parent and you're getting tired of hearing the same words coming out of your mouth over and over again, pull up a thesaurus on your phone and find different words to get your point across. If you've run out of ideas for playing with your kids, do a game exchange with a fellow family—you loan them your oft-used board games and they loan you theirs, and suddenly a whole new world of playtime is introduced to both families, absolutely free.

If you always read mysteries, pick up a nonfiction book about a subject you like. If your literary go-to is fiction, try reading a biography of someone you admire. Same goes for TV shows—if you find that all you're watching are crime dramas, take a break from that and watch a silly comedy just to get out of your usual entertainment routine.

You can change up your workout too! If you're a devotee of yoga, take a day to go swimming instead. If your usual machine of choice is the treadmill, try the rower or experiment with getting your heart rate up by punching a heavy bag.

Try changing up your cooking. When we're super busy we can get stuck in making the same ten or fifteen meals over and over again. So, look to other cuisines, take a specific cooking class, play "Chopped" with ingredients from your own pantry, and experiment with spices and techniques you might not have used before. There are thousands of recipes and tutorials online if you've always wanted to try making your own authentic Italian cannoli or Korean bibimbap. We recently started growing our own herbs and making pasta from scratch, and while neither of these are particularly difficult, they are a nice change from our usual culinary routine.

These are just a few suggestions to help get you out of a rut if you find yourself getting tired of the same-old activities day after day. Sometimes just changing one thing about your regular routine can bring happy and unexpected things into your life that will forge a new path of joy that leaves your humdrum monotony behind.

The Magic and Enchantment of Collective Joy

One of the best experiences of collective joy I have ever witnessed still makes me laugh out loud, and the memory of it still has the power to fill me up with effervescent happiness.

It was the last day of my son's high school football team's trip to Disneyworld. We were all waiting exhaustedly for the airport buses to pick us up, and after four days of non-stop activity, people were hot, tired, and grumpy that the special time was coming to an end. Enter the well-trained, happiness-infused Disney employee to the rescue! Upon seeing all of the boys sitting around with unhappy faces, she put on some line dance music and invited everyone up to dance. At first only a few boys got up, but as the first song progressed, more and more of the kids jumped in, encouraged by their enthusiastic teammates. Before long everyone was smiling and laughing and not bothered at all by the wait time. She kept playing song after song and they all kept dancing, getting more into it with every step. If a boy didn't know the moves, a buddy took him aside and broke it down until he got it. When a new song started, you could hear whoops of excitement and cries of "This one's my favorite!" A crowd gathered to watch, and you could see the absolute delight on the people's faces as they saw (and started filming) the thirty or so giant teen-aged football players clapping, twirling, kicking, stomping, and laughing as they performed these dances together. The whole scene brought as much joy to the spectators as it did to the participants. It is one of those special memories that I keep tucked away in my heart as one of those perfect moments where time stops as you step back and take in the magic of what is going on around you. Unplanned, unrehearsed, just a bunch of human beings sharing an experience of collective joy. There's really nothing else like it.

It's the same feeling you get when you're at a professional baseball game. You start out as an individual, sitting in your own seat, watching, talking, eating, thinking about the traffic on the way home ... when all of a sudden, a player hits a home run. Instantaneously, tens of thousands of people, including yourself, simultaneously rise to their feet, raise their arms in the air, and cheer wildly. For those few moments everyone is transported to another plane *together*, which is what makes it so magical and spiritually fulfilling

Why does this happen? I think it's because it's human nature to want to belong to part of something bigger than our own individual selves. It's why people who may have differing political and religious views stand together as a nation when their national anthem is played. It's also why fraternities, sororities, clubs, and social organizations exist.

I have not studied anthropology, so I have no scientific basis for why most humans and/or animals have a pack-like mentality, but I would assume it goes back to the survivalist concept of there being safety from predators in numbers. And for anyone who has ever eaten a piece of their own birthday cake alone, I believe this quote rings true:

Joy multiplies when it is shared among friends,
but grief diminishes with every division. That is life.
—R.A. Salvatore

This is why families gather to share in the collective joy of weddings and births, and also why they gather to share in the grief of funerals. This is why when something wonderful happens (an engagement, a job promotion, a pregnancy or adoption) people share the news through announcements and usually have parties to celebrate them. There is something truly precious about members of the human race coming together to encourage and congratulate one another, and that act of coming together takes the event or occurrence to a higher, more exciting, and happier level

I think we need more collective joy experiences in our lives. The world we're living in can be very divisive, and with the saturation and infiltration of social media onto just about every aspect of what we do, there is a lot more time spent focusing on our differences (and proclaiming them at every chance) than on our similarities. There is a lot less collectivity overall, and it's the beautiful "coming together" part of most experiences that make them so much more fun and enjoyable.

Why are flash mobs so popular—both to the participants and to the passersby who film them and post them later? Because it is a bunch of individuals who are fully aligned for the common purpose of doing something fun TOGETHER. People joining together—to dance, to worship, to play, to sing, to walk or run for a cause, to witness a sporting event, to celebrate, to learn, and to create, can be a very powerful and inspiring thing in our lives. It also elevates the joy of the occasion higher than we could have imagined.

So, I encourage you all, for your next birthday, have a party or at least a get-together. Invite your neighbors over for a potluck the day after Halloween and exchange your leftover candy. Go to a game for your local triple or double A baseball team and cheer along with a bunch of strangers whom you would never meet otherwise. Or join one of the thousands of Meetup groups out there to share some collective creativity doing something you're passionate about. As has been said, "No man is an island" and "It takes a village." We all need help from others at times, but even more than that, when we share our joys and sorrows it makes them more joyful and easier to bear.

In difficult times, try to surround yourself with others for support. In happy times, try to surround yourself with people who can be happy with you. Loneliness is not an option for any of us, *unless we choose it*. SHARE YOURSELF with others. Actively participate in collective joy, and you'll end up with gleeful memories that you can draw on whenever you need a reminder of the good that can happen when people choose to join together as one.

Happiness is not something ready-made.

It comes from your own actions.

—THE DALAI LAMA

Stop Dusting Your Pipes

Some years ago, I met a woman who regularly dusted her pipes. That's not a metaphor; every few weeks she would go into the little room with the water heater and the piping and duct work in her house and clean off every surface in there. She even had a stepladder propped up against the wall for just that purpose.

In all of the places I have lived during my lifetime I can honestly say that not once, even for a millisecond, has it ever occurred to me to dust my pipes. And considering that every other person whom I have told about this particular practice has responded, "She does WHAT?!" I'm guessing that it hasn't occurred to most other people either.

It became very apparent (after additional things she told me and showed me in her home) that this person suffers from severe OCD, which completely explains the compulsive pipe dusting. But that repeated, useless act made me think about the countless hours so many of us spend doing meaningless things or being slaves to our unhealthy impulses. We may not physically dust our pipes, but what else do we do that we really don't need to?

In other words, what is our version of dusting our pipes? Is it watching video after video on YouTube instead of creating something artistic ourselves? Is it endlessly scrolling Facebook or Instagram, looking at other people having a good time while we're sitting home alone at the computer? Is it doing that scrolling while feeling jealous of those other people's high-light reels and negating our own lives and accomplishments by comparison? Is it constantly worrying about every single thing we put into our mouths because of the caloric or carb or fat content? Is it constantly thinking about the past and how we were wronged or hurt by someone? Is it the continual play-ing of the tape in our head that tells us we're not good enough, pretty enough, smart enough, capable enough, thin enough, talented enough, insert-whatever-self-deprecating-word-here enough to really go after our dreams and try to make them a reality?

There are so many ways that we regularly "dust our pipes," and none of them are worthy of our time and effort. They are all time-wasting, joy-sucking, and nonsensical things to do with our time. As bizarre as it is to think of someone climbing up on a ladder every few weeks to dust her pipes, it's likewise as crazy to spend precious moments of our days focusing on things that don't matter even a little bit.

I encourage you to make the choice to stop doing whatever it is that equates to the inanity of dusting your pipes. Choose instead to spend your time doing activities that make you happy and fill up your spirit. The pipes will always be there, but they do not, I repeat, DO NOT require your attention. Only the marvelousness that is *you*, does.

Help Others

When you help someone up a hill
you find yourself closer to the top.
—Brownie Wise

Helping others is a recurring theme throughout this book. Why? Because I have found it to be a foolproof way of choosing happiness. When you lift someone else up, you get lifted up at the same time. Every time.

Studies have shown that when we help someone else, our brain releases oxytocin—the "feel good" hormone—so it doesn't just lift our spirits emotionally, it makes us feel better on a chemical level. Studies have also shown that people witnessing someone helping someone else also raises the oxytocin levels in *their* brains, which means that when you go outside of yourself to help someone else, they feel good, you feel good, and anyone else in the vicinity ALSO feels good.

This seems like such a simple cure-all for everything, doesn't it?

The other thing that helping someone else does for us is it gets us out of our own heads. We get the wonderful opportunity to focus on something besides what we're dealing with mentally, and I know I can speak for myself that a break from that can be a welcome and necessary reprieve. Helping someone else can also put our own lives into sharp perspective and remind us to be grateful for what we have. It only takes a few minutes of volunteering at a food bank or a soup kitchen to kick our gratitude into gear for the food and shelter that we enjoy (and possibly take for granted) every day.

So often we are taught, especially in the workplace, that if we help someone else we will be damaging our own chances for advancement. I believe the opposite is true. I myself have had people sabotage my work efforts and try to cut me down on both professional and personal levels. Those people did get ahead in the short term, but over time, co-workers and su-pervisors saw their self-centered and egocentric behavior, and none of them ended up getting the high positions they wanted in their careers. As a supervisor myself, I saw the interactions of my staff—and the employees who stood out to me were the ones who stayed late to help their colleagues finish a proj-ect, who brought coffee and treats to boost exhausted people's spirits, and who gave credit to their entire team instead of making sure their names were front and center on completed tasks. Those were the people who got the promotions, not the people who were only looking out for themselves.

There are so many ways to help others, in big ways, in small ways, and in so many ways in-between. Wouldn't we all like to live in a world where people consistently help each other up instead of tearing one another down? Wouldn't we like to be the people who attempt to create that world around us as much as we can?

I encourage you to do your part in creating the world you want to live in; where we all go out of our way to help others without thinking about how it might benefit ourselves, even though with regard to our own happiness it always does.

When you have a

really difficult decision to make:

Flip a coin.

It doesn't matter how it lands.

Your answer will come when you realize

how you are hoping it will land

on its way down.

Keep a Happiness Journal

What a brilliant idea. This is from Michele M. Cook's website,
www.michelesfindinghappiness.com.

What Is a Happiness Journal?

A happiness journal is simply a record of the things that
make you happy each day. It doesn't have to be a physically
written journal, it can be an electronic journal, a photo
journal, or a music journal. Your learning style will determine what type of happiness journal will suit you the best.

For me, it is a combination of photos and a physically
written journal. This works for me because I love taking
pictures and I love the act of putting a pen to paper and
writing something down. What works for you may be different; maybe you want to use just a photo journal, maybe
a music and electronic journal. The important thing here
is that you find what works for you, as this will help you
get into a rhythm of using it every day. Here are a few
types of journals that you could try. If more than one
sounds interesting to you, don't be afraid to try and combine a few types.

*Michele Cook, "How to Start a Happiness Journal," https://michelesfinding
happiness.com/2016/08/01/start-happiness-journal/, August 1, 2016.

- Written journal. A book of blank pages that you use a pen to write things down.
- Electronic journal. Any type of document system that you can write with. Google docs, Notepad, Microsoft Word all work. This is also the easiest to combine with pictures or music.
- Photo journal. Tell your story through pictures with minimal writing. You might want to add a few captions here and there so when you review your journal, you remember why you took a picture of that rock.
- Music journal. Use songs or snippets of songs to tell your happiness story. Again, you might want to add a caption so you remember why you saved the chorus to "Girls Just Wanna Have Fun."

Why Should I Start a Happiness Journal?

Well, to make you happy, of course. Happiness journals are designed to make you think about your happiness throughout the day. After doing this for a few days, you will start to pay more attention to the happier things of your day, and less attention will be focused on the not so happy things. The longer you use a happiness journal the better your results will be. As you go through your days, you will start looking for those happy moments and think, "That is going in the journal tonight!"

Creating a happiness journal creates a worldview shift. A happiness journal is not going to stop bad things from happening in our lives, but it will help the way we see and deal with them. We spend plenty of time worrying about the bad things in life. A happiness journal adds balance, so we spend some time looking at the good things too.

What Should I Put in My Journal?

What you put in the journal each day is up to you, but the idea is to put at least one thing per day in the journal that makes you happy. As you go throughout your day, take note of things that make you happy in one way or another. Here are a few ideas on how you can put your journal together.

- **Take a picture.** Each day take a picture of something that makes you happy. In the evening, print it or add it to an electronic journal with a little caption about why it made you happy.
- **Try a bullet journal.** For those of us who are all about the facts, a bullet journal can work great. Use three bullet points per day and write a short sentence or two about what made you happy that day.
- **Take notes.** During the day, when something makes you happy, make a little note somewhere. At the end of the day, pull all of your notes together and pick the one that made you the happiest. If you can't decide, there are really no rules here, use more than one!

Your happiness journal is yours; you decide what goes into it and what doesn't. The important part of a happiness journal is that you put something in it every day.

Even on your worst day, you should try to find one act of kindness that someone did for you, one smile or one scene that made your mood lift ever so slightly.

... A happiness journal can shift your focus from all of the drama and doldrums of everyday life to the smiles and the silliness of everyday life. ...

... The best part is going back and looking at each page and remembering all those little things that made you happy.

Have fun with this! Enjoy creating this great tool for your Happiness Toolbox!

When Times Are Bleak, Do Something!

A few years ago my husband left his job to start his own company. He had been beyond miserable for too long and based on some promising information from potential clients he took an enormous leap of faith to finally become his own boss. Within about three months he was back to his happy self and there was a lightness to his spirit that hadn't been there for some time. Everything was great!

As life has a tendency to throw us curve balls sometimes, the main clients that he had secured to start the business all fell through at once, and we were left with a dearth of income. With one kid in college and one about to start in less than a year, plus our mortgage, electric bill, car payments, and our other regular expenses looming, we were both worried about our immediate financial future. To make matters worse, I had left my job a few months earlier, which didn't bring in a ton of money but was great for incidentals and provided a cushion if we needed it.

After a few sleepless nights of worrying incessantly, I finally decided that I had to DO SOMETHING. Being passive about this situation was not going to help anything, and while I didn't have another job yet, I felt like sure that I could at least do something, anything, to contribute and help in some way. So I dug out my old Tightwad Gazette book (from our newlywed days) and dove in.

First I went through our stuff with a critical eye and sold some of it on eBay and at consignment shops. I didn't make much from those endeavors, but I felt good that I was at least bringing in a small amount of money for things that were just gathering dust anyway. I also tried to figure out creative ways to cut down on daily expenses. Since I like to cook, I started in the kitchen.

I started creating food items that were far cheaper to make than to buy. For example, I started making my own pizza dough. Flour and yeast are inexpensive, and the great thing about making dough from scratch is that everyone can make it to their own liking. Thin crust, thick crust, covered in Parmesan cheese, we tried them all. Making our own pizzas, especially when topped with fresh vegetables, cut down the cost immensely and was far healthier than our usual takeout options. I also started making my own salad dressing and croutons, which were so much fresher and better than anything from a store. All of our baked goods were homemade (and who doesn't prefer freshly baked chocolate chip cookies to anything you'd find in a package?), as well as hummus, marinara sauce, granola, and a plethora of other things. Holiday gifts that year were applesauce and peach butter that I made and canned from our backyard fruit trees.

The list goes on and on, but the point is, instead of worrying about things, I MADE THE CONSCIOUS CHOICE TO DO SOMETHING ABOUT THEM. Ultimately my pioneer ways probably didn't save us a significant amount of money, but it was a great alternative to getting stressed about our financial situation.

My advice to you is, for whatever situation you're in that's bringing you down, DO SOMETHING! If you're lonely, join a Meetup or a singles group. If you're unhappy at your work, make a concerted effort to find something new that will fulfill you. If you're upset about your past and living inside your own head, find a therapist or support group that can help you. Whatever it is, just DO SOMETHING. It might end up solving the problem, but even if it doesn't, you can at least know that you did more than just passively settle for your current lot in life.

Make the choice. Choose action over inaction, proactivity over passivity, positivity over negativity, and hope over fear. In this way, you'll be choosing happiness no matter what curve ball life throws at you next.

When Times Are Bleak for Others, Do Something!

Also known as Help Others, Part Two.

I'm one of those people who is first in line at someone's house with a meal when I've heard that they have lost a loved one. I've been known to bring chicken soup to people's homes when they are sick, and nothing makes me happier than sending gifts and encouragement to people when they are having a hard time. It's just part of my makeup—always has been, always will be.

The recipients of my intended-to-be-helpful acts react with mixed responses. Some are happy, excited, and grateful. (I had someone burst into tears post-surgery when I dropped off a meal at her house because at the age of forty-five no one had ever cooked anything for her before.) Some are angry, offended, and annoyed. (I've heard all manner of "You're crazy!" and "I didn't ask for this!" and "This is terrible! I can never pay you back for this." Which is absolutely not the point by the way.) Some are just plain bewildered. (When I dropped off a meal for a colleague upon hearing that her mother had passed away, her husband asked me, "What is this for? Do you think we don't know how to cook?")

Sigh.

The two most interesting responses are what I want to talk about though. Twice in my life, both of them recently, I heard from people I've sent things to when I've heard about their dire cancer diagnoses.

One person said, "This is great. Everyone else asks us, 'What can I do?' but you just jump in and DO."

The other one said, "Thank you for what you sent. Most people shy away when they hear about me and what's going on, but you decided to jump in and do something instead of turning away. That means the world to me."

The same words echoed by two different people. "Jump in," and "Do something."

It honestly would never occur to me NOT to, but again, this is just part of who I am. I'm not saying this to pat myself on the back or tout my giving instincts—honestly, I'm not. I'm just saying that for me it's kind of a reflex and it reflects the way I was raised. So even though I've received my share of negative feedback with regard to doing these things, it's not something that I can "not do," if that makes sense.

I think it's because even though I can't do anything to fix the situation, it's something I CAN DO to hopefully at least make the situation a little easier to bear.

On a more global level, if you're upset by the state of the world, maybe it would help to do something, even something small, just to make you feel like you're contributing to a solution in some way. Volunteer at a food bank, build homes with Habitat for Humanity, teach a class at a homeless shelter or at a Boys and Girls Club—the list of ways that you can help is endless. Using whatever talents and strengths you have to do something to help the situation that is keeping you up at night can go a long way in your choosing happiness journey.

RESOURCES

Habitat for Humanity, www.habitat.org

Homeless Shelters, www.homelessshelterdirectory.org

Boys and Girls Clubs of America, www.bgca.org

Best Buddies, www.bestbuddies.org

Special Olympics, www.specialolympics.org

AmeriCorps, www.nationalservice.gov/program/americorps

Peace Corps, www.peacecorps.gov

Talk Less, Listen More

If I had my life to live over
I would have talked less and listened more.
—Erma Bombeck

So, I'm currently on day three of complete laryngitis. I'm not hoarse, I'm not raspy—when I try to speak or make any kind of sound at all, literally nothing comes out. All I keep thinking about is Ariel in *The Little Mermaid* when Ursula tells her "That's right sweet cakes, no talking, no singing, zip."

This has been surprisingly difficult for me. I do not consider myself a "talker," although I do enjoy good conversations. For the past six years or so I have made a conscious effort to talk less and listen more, and to be a considerate and conscientious listener. I started paying attention to my listening vs. talking ratio after reading Erma Bombeck's quote and especially after hearing a college student from a different country explain the things that he didn't like about living in America. His main complaint was that Americans don't really listen, but rather pretend to listen during a conversation, all the while planning what they are going to say next. As the other person finishes what they had to say or sometimes even before that (apparently Americans are well known for interrupting others), the American jumps in with his or her opinion or advice on the matter, making it abundantly clear that what they had to say was much more important than the original speaker's words.

Now of course I'm not saying that every person does this, nor is this rather rude habit reserved solely for Americans. But as I've been unable to speak for the past three days it has made me realize how often I open my mouth when there's simply no need to. It's not urgently necessary to fill silence all the time; in fact, there can be something nice about two people sitting together, enjoying the stillness and peace that comes with quiet moments shared.

This lapse in talking has also made me realize that as much as I don't think I'm one of those "I'm not really listening but instead planning what I'm about to say" people, at times I actually am. Especially when someone is talking about something that I have a particular interest in or opinion about. This was a disappointing realization, but a necessary one for me, because I honestly do not want to be that kind of person, in any situation. For the past few days I have been forced to listen; really listen, to others, and pause before reacting in the only ways that I currently can—a thumbs up, a nod, a smile, etc., because I am completely unable to plan ahead to respond in any other way. An excellent learning experience for sure.

I also believe that the whole "Talk Less ... Listen More" concept applies to online commenting as well. I personally never comment on anything online, but for the millions of people who get some satisfaction about typing their (usually negative) opinions online for anyone and everyone to see, I have to wonder if they might have happier and more truly fulfilling lives if they spent less time "talking" in front of a computer screen to no one, and more time engaging with real people and real-life experiences. I mean, has anyone said on their deathbed, "I wish I had trolled more people on the Internet and spewed more negativity out into the world?"

I'm choosing to use this slightly difficult and inconvenient time as a lesson in talking less and listening more, and I intend to carry on this practice once my voice returns. It's a great reminder that when someone else has the floor it's not about me. I'll get my turn. I can be patient. I can realize that it's not always all about what I have to say. It also takes the pressure off of me feeling like I *must* say something to fill the silence or to add my two cents even when it wasn't asked for. And that's definitely a happy choice for me.

Keep Household Clutter under Control

There is no need for me to go through the hows and whys of decluttering here. There are plenty of books, articles, and (very fun and interesting) TV shows dedicated to this subject. What I will throw in are my two cents on "stuff" and decluttering in general.

I am a big believer in the concepts that organizational gurus like Marie Kondo and Peter Walsh proselytize: Things are just things, keep something only if it sparks joy, and as things accumulate we should periodically go through our possessions and give away or throw out the things that we don't use and don't need.

Because we have moved across the country a few times, we have done a massive purge each time, getting rid of unnecessary things and deciding if we wanted to begin our new chapter with or without this item or that item. We have also lost some things in moves—nothing of huge monetary or sentimental value, thankfully—but experiencing that tangible loss helps us to remember the fallibility of material possessions and reminds us of what we can often live happily without.

Case in point: when we first moved to where we currently live, the moving truck got delayed and wasn't going to arrive until five to seven days after we got to our rental place. All we had with us were a few bags of clothing and essentials we had been using on the cross-country drive. To make things even more difficult, our two kids were starting school the following day (unbeknownst to us until we arrived) and they didn't even have a pencil with which to begin their school year.

So along with school supplies, we set about getting the things we needed to tide us over until our belongings arrived. We were very thoughtful about what to purchase, since we wanted to double up as little as possible. We ended up with one bath towel for each of us, some air mattresses and sheets (thankfully we already had our pillows), a shower curtain and a few trash cans. Our kitchen supplies consisted of one frying pan, one pot, one mixing bowl, one mixing spoon, one knife, one cutting board, four plates, four sets of utensils, one baking tray, and one set of dish towels and oven mitts. Guess what we found out?

We actually need very little to maintain a happy existence. Guess what else we found out?

Dirty dishes didn't pile up in the sink because we had to wash everything immediately for the next meal. Laundry didn't pile up and become mountainous because we didn't have that many clothes to wash. It was really easy to find things because there weren't other things getting in the way. That first week of living with only a few necessities had a noticeable, comfortable, and beautiful simplicity to it.

It was also fun to sleep on air mattresses on the floor and crowd around the tiny bistro table set for dinner. The kids did their homework lying on the living room floor, and we made a "sofa" by piling up blankets and jackets from the car. We had a great time "camping" for that first week in a new place, and I often remember the joy of living simply with the few possessions we owned, instead of our many possessions own-ing us.

Now, I'm not saying that I would like to live that way all the time. I love my various kitchen gadgets and tables covered in framed family photographs. But it's nice to know that none of us needs a lot of stuff to create and live a happy life.

One more thing, and this may be a controversial thing to say, but it's just my opinion, take it or leave it with what works for you and your lifestyle.

No one needs a storage unit.

If you have so much extraneous stuff you are not using on a regular basis, that you are paying money on a monthly basis to store and NOT USE, then to me, that is a waste of money and space. I knew someone who had to go through her deceased mother's two storage units of random stuff—old clothes, por-celain figurines, half-finished sewing projects and mountains of fabric and craft supplies, long unneeded paperwork and files, and sets upon sets of never-used dishware that she was holding onto for other family members. My friend said that not only had there been tens of thousands of dollars spent over the last twenty years to store it all, but when she took a week off of work to painstakingly go through it to see what was salvageable, much of it had been ruined by mold, dirt, animals and their waste. She even found a rat carcass among some of the clothes, which, if you think about it, they were paying good money to keep there.

I know that people keep storage units for various reasons, and I would never tell anyone how or where to keep their stuff. But I am saying that to choose happiness sometimes we have to take a good hard look at our lives and what may be getting in the way of us being able to make that choice. Oftentimes excessive clutter and too many material possessions can be real roadblocks to the happy and less stressed lives that we want. Conquering our clutter and our attachment to material things can be a huge step toward that, and it helps to remember that no tangible thing can ever fill an empty place inside our hearts, nor can it ever show us warmth, affection, approval, or love. Some things can make us happy, for sure, and they are essential in helping us to fulfill the dreams we have for ourselves, but not one material thing can ever, nor will ever, cause true, long-lasting happiness.

> *Clutter is a stealer of joy and contentment.*
> *Your home should breathe happiness into your family's*
> *story, not slowly suck the life out of you.*
> —Melissa Michaels,
> author of *Make Room for What You Love*

RESOURCES

It's All Too Much: An Easy Plan for Living a Richer Life with Less Stuff, by Peter Walsh

Let It Go: Downsizing Your Way to a Richer, Happier Life, by Peter Walsh

Lighten Up: Love What You Have, Have What You Need, Be Happier with Less, by Peter Walsh

The Life-Changing Magic of Tidying Up: The Japanese Art of Decluttering and Organizing, by Marie Kondo

Spark Joy: An Illustrated Master Class on the Art of Organizing and Tidying Up (companion to *The Life Changing Magic of Tidying Up*), by Marie Kondo

Tidying Up with Marie Kondo, www.netflix.com (I love this show!)

The only reason you are happy

is because you choose to be happy.

Happiness is a choice

and so is suffering.

—MIGUEL ANGEL RUIZ

Change the Station

So I was driving along today, happily and contentedly, when an old song came on the radio. It was a song that brought back some particularly painful memories, and as I listened, I felt myself reliving all of those old feelings. All of a sudden I was feeling sad, discouraged, bummed out, and in a matter of seconds my entire outlook and demeanor changed. My previously happy mood took a nosedive and I found myself almost beginning to cry right there in the car.

At that moment I heard a little voice inside my head that said, "You know, you can change the station."

Change the station. Right! I didn't have to sit there feeling miserable listening to that stupid song, I had the power to change the station! The song and the feelings that it brought back did NOT have power over me—I had power over them—and I didn't have to succumb to them and keep on suffering.

Armed with this newfound wisdom, I reached over, pressed a little button, and the song was instantly replaced by a happy, upbeat song, and my good mood returned. How about that!

And that got me thinking . . . how often do we NOT change the station in our lives? How many times do we get pulled down by the past, or find ourselves stuck in a rut, or feel hopeless that we can't change anything about our current situation? We think that we are powerless over our own thoughts, which, when you think about it, is absurd. All we have to do is change the station in our minds.

We can't expect anyone else to do it for us. It's up to us to *choose* to change what we don't like about our lives. Like those "friends" who let us down on a regular basis, or that co-worker who is constantly taking advantage of our good nature and work ethic, or those memories that send us spiraling downward instead of lifting us up—we don't have to get stuck in those anymore. We don't have to continue on in relationships that don't make us happy or feed our souls. We don't have to say "yes" to every single person's request of us. We are not stuck where we think we are, regardless of our circumstances.

Most importantly though, I think we need to change the station when it comes to what we tell ourselves. There's that little voice in our heads that tells us we're not good enough, or that we'll never get it all accomplished, or that it's pointless to even try because it's not going to work out anyway. It also pipes up to remind us that happiness means the other shoe will drop at any minute, and that it's foolish to have high hopes and dreams for ourselves. Oftentimes these words were spoken originally by someone else but we have made them our own, and we cling to them as the absolute truth. This particular station needs to be turned off completely, replaced by presets that applaud our successes, foster joy and optimism, and encourage us in our pursuits and endeavors. Let these be the ones we go to when we look in the mirror or talk to others or think about trying something new.

We don't need to be stuck listening to the same old songs anymore. We can just change the station. And do you know what happens when we do that? We find a whole bunch of new songs that we get to sing along to and enjoy.

Smile!

… even when you might not feel like smiling.

The following are excerpts from a report at nbcnews.com, written by journalist Nicole Spector. *

Ever had someone tell you to cheer up and smile? It's probably not the most welcomed advice, especially when you're feeling sick, tired or just plain down in the dumps. But there's actually a good reason to turn that frown upside down. … Science has shown that … smiling can lift your mood, lower stress, boost your immune system and possibly even prolong your life.

It's a pretty backwards idea, isn't it? Happiness is what makes us smile; how can the reverse also be true? The fact is, as Dr. Isha Gupta, a neurologist from IGEA Brain and Spine, explains, a smile spurs a chemical reaction in the brain, releasing certain hormones including dopamine and serotonin. "Dopamine increases our feelings of happiness. Serotonin release is associated with reduced stress. Low levels of serotonin are associated with depression and aggression," says Dr. Gupta. "Low levels of dopamine are also associated with depression."

*Nicole Spector, "Smiling Can Trick Your Brain into Happiness—and Boost Your Health," https://www.nbcnews.com/better/health/smiling-can-trick-your-brain-happiness-boost-your-health-ncna822591, updated on January 9, 2018.

...Smiling can trick your brain into believing you're happy, which can then spur actual feelings of happiness. But it doesn't end there. Dr. Murray Grossan, an ENT-otolaryngologist in Los Angeles, points to the science of psychoneuroimmunology (the study of how the brain is connected to the immune system), asserting that it has been shown "over and over again" that depression weakens your immune system, while happiness ... has been shown to boost our body's resistance.

"What's crazy is that just the physical act of smiling can make a difference in building your immunity," says Dr. Grossan. "When you smile, the brain sees the muscle activity and assumes that humor is happening."

[T]he brain ... doesn't bother to sort out whether you're smiling because you're genuinely joyous, or because you're just pretending.

"Even forcing a fake smile can legitimately reduce stress and lower your heart rate," adds Dr. Sivan Finkel, a cosmetic dentist at NYC's The Dental Parlour. "A study performed by a group at the University of Cardiff in Wales found that people who could not frown due to botox injections were happier on average than those who could frown."

And there are plenty more studies out there to make you smile. ... Researchers at the University of Kansas published findings that smiling helps reduce the body's response to stress and lower heart rate in tense situations; another study linked smiling to lower blood pressure, while yet another suggests that smiling leads to longevity.

Additionally, when traveling there is one thing that one realizes quite fast: a smile can change everything.

It can open doors and the hearts of other people whose culture you do not even know. A smile is the most international language that everyone knows.

A smile is also something that is easy to pass on. Much like yawning, smiling is contagious. ... A smile's contagion is so potent that we may even be able to catch one from ourselves. Dr. Ritzo recommends smiling at yourself in the mirror, an act she says not only triggers our mirror neurons but can also help us calm down and re-center if we're feeling low or anxious.

It turns out there's solid evidence that smiling can do us a world of good. Since researching this piece I've been conducting my own little smile experiments. I tried smiling when I tensed up in traffic yesterday, and again during a rigorous workout and then today when I woke up with a headache. I found that it feels completely incongruous to smile when I'm tense or tired, and there's a strange sense of departing a comfort zone. But I have to admit, instantly I was calmer, less upset and, maybe just ever so slightly for a second, smiling made me feel happy.

Me again.

I think it's so cool that the simple act of making ourselves smile, even when we're not feeling particularly happy, sends the signals to our brains that happiness is occurring, and it responds accordingly, which in turn makes us feel happy. It's such a simple thing, and yet it can be incredibly powerful when we need it to be.

Eat the Birthday Cake

A party without cake is just a meeting.
—Julia Child

Do you know what I believe to be one of life's greatest pleasures? Birthday cake! I don't care if it comes from the supermarket, or a fancy bakery, or if it's homemade (my favorite), it's all good and it's all worthy of being eaten.

Why? Because it's a tangible way of celebrating someone on a special day, and it's a vital part of any milestone celebration. There's a reason why the party frivolity comes to a halt and everyone gathers around to watch the candles get blown out and serenade the person of honor. There's a reason why there's a whole cake-cutting ceremony at a wedding. And there's a reason why there are at least a dozen shows on television expressly geared toward showcasing the art of cake decorating.

Having a cake at a celebration is important. We may not know why it's important, but it is.

I attended a nutrition workshop many years ago where the leader spent a good 45 minutes extolling the merits of a vegetarian-leaning-toward-vegan lifestyle. She spoke vehemently about the evils of sugar and salt in the American diet and gave us tips about how to utilize natural spices and the healing virtues of many of them. Then, right toward the end, she said something that has stayed with me to this day. She said:

"No matter what kind of diet you're on, when it's your child's birthday, EAT THE BIRTHDAY CAKE!"

What? Here she was, telling all of us what NOT to eat, and pretty much every one of those things (sugar, fat, white flour) are the essential ingredients in a birthday cake. She went on to explain:

"No matter what kind of diet you're following, a slice of birthday cake one or two times a year is not going to make a difference in your health journey one way or another. But what WILL make a difference is what you're communicating to your child in that moment."

In her opinion, if you choose to refuse the birthday cake at your child's birthday party, your actions are saying to him or her, "My 'stuff' is more important than your 'stuff.' My strict adherence to making sure I look a certain way and monitoring everything I put into my mouth is more important than sharing in the joy of this celebration honoring you." And while most kids won't notice if you ARE eating birthday cake at their birthday party, they will most definitely notice if you ARE NOT.

Interesting food for thought, no?

All puns aside, I believe what she said is one hundred percent true. I also believe that part of celebrating with other people includes partaking of the customary food that is offered and shared. Also, in those special moments of joy and laudation, I think we do ourselves a disservice by not allowing ourselves to truly immerse ourselves in the happiness and exaltation of a sacred bit of time and space that will never happen again. Your child only has one birthday per year and each celebration is ancient history by the time the next one rolls around. The same goes for other family members and friends whose parties you will hopefully be lucky enough to be invited to and to attend.

In order for us to make the conscious choice to really choose happiness in our lives, I think that one way is to eat the birthday cake, whenever we get the chance. It reminds us that life is to be celebrated as often as possible, and that freely taking part in those celebrations can be uplifting and joyous for everyone in the room.

Create What Brings You Joy and Don't Ever Be Discouraged from Doing So

This is a piece I wrote for a Pennsylvania Governor's School for the Arts Alumni Publication.

A message to the artists out there:

I recently became reacquainted with a friend from my childhood. I also reconnected with his mother, and I sent her some of my CDs as a way to hopefully help uplift her during her extremely courageous battle with cancer. A few weeks ago she lost that battle, and today the friend reached out to tell me that when he went back to his mom's house, he popped open the CD player in her kitchen (the one that she always played, he said) and one of my CDs was in there. He thanked me for providing her with some joy and hope through my music, especially during the last few months when things got really difficult.

This brought me to tears and touched me deeply because it reminded me of why we artists do what we do. Very few of us will ever be famous and most of us will never even be able to make a living by our craft. But that should never discourage us or make us think that what we create isn't worthwhile. Awards and applause are fun, and we all want to be recognized for our work and feel like it's making a difference in some way. But just because we haven't sold a million albums or had our artwork shown in a gallery or have a book on a bestseller list **does not mean that our art isn't appreciated, meaningful, or valuable.**

So many musicians' and artists' talents were never acknowledged during their lifetimes, and it was only decades (or in some cases centuries) later that their genius was given the renown it was due. So why did they continue pursuing their art? For the same reason that we all do. Because it's what we were put on this Earth to do. That impulse inside of us that needs to create something artistic should never be squelched; in fact, it needs to be honored and acted upon, even if nobody ever sees what we've created. *It's the creating that matters.* It's also important to remember that for the people who do see or hear our artistic endeavors, it could have a life-changing positive impact on them that we may never know about.

Art in its many forms—painting, music, dance, film, sculpture, photography, poetry, theater, prose, and more—has the ability to cut through the noise in a person's mind and bring them serenity, beauty, hope, and encouragement. There's a reason why people go to museums to be inspired or listen to music when they work out. The arts have such significant importance in the world, and I know that when I see or hear a miraculous piece of art I can be transported to a place where the unimaginable becomes possible.

So, to my fellow artists I want to say, keep on doing what you were born to do. While you may not receive the kudos or the compensation that you dream of, you need to keep contributing the art that only you can produce in your own inimitable way. When you create and put forth the art that is inside of you, that alone makes you a successful artist.

> *The purpose of art is nothing less than*
> *the upliftment of the human spirit.*
> —Pope John Paul II

Keep on lifting up those human spirits—we need you now more than ever.

—Rachel Cole
October 9, 2020

Unconditional Happiness

I recently heard about a concept called "Unconditional Happiness." The person talking about it said that when she finally learned to let go of anger and focus instead on being unconditionally happy, it saved her life.

I started thinking about this concept, and my first thought was, "Is this even possible? Can a person really be unconditionally happy all the time? Especially when you look at what's going on in the world and how people are treating each other?"

I thought for a few more minutes about it, and my answer became a resounding YES! It's completely possible! I don't think it means that we are blithely skipping around in our lives surrounded by rainbows and unicorns or being "checked out" in a constant state of ignorance and elation. But I DO think it's possible to make the choice to focus on the good and to keep ourselves as happy as we can regardless of what is happening outside of ourselves, which is often completely out of our control.

I look at it this way: What is unconditional love? It's loving someone with our full hearts and minds and souls **no matter what**. It doesn't matter what they say, what they do, or what mood they are in at a given time. We are going to love them without condition, without strings attached, and without demanding or expecting anything in return. I believe we can apply the same properties to unconditional happiness. We can say that we are going to be happy regardless of what someone says to us, how someone acts toward us, or whatever mood we happen to be in. **It also means that I choose to find happiness and positivity in situations, no matter what else is going on around me.**

Take a traffic jam—this is the worst, right? I have to be somewhere, I'm already running late, now I'm stuck in bumper to bumper traffic, which means now I will most definitely be late and UGH! Why does this always happen to me? I can't believe this is happening NOW! ARGH!

My blood pressure is rising just thinking about this scenario.

How do we react if we're practicing unconditional happiness? We first put the situation into perspective and recognize that while it's not ideal, it's also not the end of the world. No one is hurt, no one is sick, all that's really going on is that we're a little inconvenienced and things aren't going exactly according to the original plan. Secondly, we take a moment to be grateful that we weren't the ones in the accident that caused the backup, or if it's because of construction, we can be very glad and grateful that we're not the ones who have to be outside in the blistering heat or freezing cold, completely exposed to the elements for eight hours a day doing hard manual labor. Next, we can take the opportunity of being stuck to talk to the people in the car with us if we're not alone. We can play a fun car game or ask some Table Topic type questions to generate some insightful conversation that we'll all enjoy. If we're by ourselves in the car, we can still do the first two things, and then we can play around on the radio to find a song we like, perhaps finding a radio station that we were previously unaware of. Or we can fire up a podcast that we had been meaning to listen to but hadn't gotten around to yet. Or we can make a mental list of all of the things that we're grateful for or looking forward to, like a dream vacation or completing things on our bucket list. Take that unexpected suspended time and consciously turn it around from something annoying and frustrating into something fun and joyful.

Not to mention, has getting angry and exasperated at a situation that is completely out of your control EVER changed it one iota? Nope. So, there's really no point in getting worked up over it.

Here's another example: You have a whole day planned with the kids at an amusement park, but you wake up and it's pouring down rain. Or the place is unexpectedly closed. Or one kid wakes up with a fever and you're not going anywhere. This can be a really disappointing thing for everyone. And yes, you are allowed to rant and rave and shake your fist at the sky and bemoan your circumstances ... for about five minutes. After that, you make the choice to move on with the excited glee that comes with finding out about a snow day. That's the greatest feeling in the world, isn't it? A snow day! It's actually the same thing—your original plans were changed at the last minute, leaving your day open for something unplanned and filled with possibility.

So, you look at this turn of events like a snow day, and you fill it with the things you all like to do indoors. You bake cookies, you play board games, you put on music and dance around the living room, you have a movie marathon—which is something you'd never have time for otherwise—you make a pillow fort and climb inside with flashlights and read stories to each other. You have breakfast for dinner, you paint pictures on the windows, you finally put together the jigsaw puzzle or

Lego set that has been sitting there waiting for you to have enough time. You make the best of it, and don't focus on the fact that your original plans were thwarted by something you couldn't control.

Admittedly, these are easy fixes. But how do we continue to have unconditional happiness when the really hard things come? A friend's betrayal. The death of a loved one. A dire diagnosis.

Well, in those times we allow ourselves some measure of anger, grief, disappointment, and self-pity, but we do not allow ourselves to remain mired in that swamp for too long. We consciously pick ourselves up and focus on the good. The person we love has left us, but there are still flowers blooming in the yard, there are still ducks swimming in the pond, and we still have the gift of being alive ourselves to enjoy these things. The diagnosis is devastating, but it's also an opportunity to research treatments, to receive love and care from others, and to treasure each day as it comes. The friend who pulled the rug out from under us is not a person beneficial to us in our journey and we were thankfully spared from something worse happening down the line. These may all sound like rationalizations, but who cares? We do not have control over the bad things that happen in our lives—all we have control over is how we deal with them. And choosing to be happy in spite of pain and loss is sometimes the only way we can prevent a spiral of darkness that can be nearly impossible to pull ourselves out of.

I'm in favor of unconditional happiness because it is a mindset that can get us through some of the most difficult times in our lives. It can also make the good times even better since we're starting out at an optimistic level of joy to begin with. And for the person who dismisses this concept as a naive and Pollyanna way to go through life, I would ask them this question:

Has anyone ever come to the end of their life and said, "I just wish my life had been more miserable?"

Choose Happiness. Make that, Choose Unconditional Happiness.

Laugh in the Rain

Today, for the first time in three and half months I went for a walk with my good friend Liz. It was wonderful to be out in the fresh air and as we embarked on our typical route, we noticed some dark, ominous looking clouds not too far off in the distance. "It'll be fine," we reassured each other. We had checked the weather, there was only a ten percent chance of rain, and we were certain that those clouds were on their way out and definitely not on their way in to where we were standing.

Well, both we and the weather predictors couldn't have been more wrong. It began drizzling when we reached our halfway mark, and about three minutes after that the sky opened up and we got caught in a deluge. We raced to put our phones safely away in pockets and waistbands, and after about five minutes of freezing driving rain, the hail began.

It was actually kind of comical. There we were, taking our first stroll together in such a long time, and we get dumped on by a flash flood complete with balls of ice pelting onto our bare skin. Rather than get annoyed or grumpy at the situation however, we kept giggling at ourselves as we pushed our bedraggled hair out of our eyes and made silly remarks like, "Good thing we put on sunscreen!" and "Someone should really come up with hailscreen!"

There was nowhere to run for cover, so we trudged on, our feet sloshing in our now saturated sneakers, trying to remember a time when we had been so fully drenched that didn't include taking a shower. When we finally reached an underpass where we could get a brief respite from the torrents, we met a similarly soaked-to-the-skin runner trying to wring out his shirt. Our eyes met and we all just laughed at the insane situation we were in, assuring each other that we were not complete dolts and we had all in fact checked the weather report before venturing out when we did.

The rain stopped shortly afterward, and my friend and I slogged home in different directions in our sopping, waterlogged shoes. As we parted, she said, "Well, we'll definitely always remember THIS walk, huh?" It was such a ridiculous situation, and one that most definitely could have been miserable. There were plenty of reasons to be upset about what had happened: The fact that we were as far away as possible from the entrance/exit when the rain started. ("Of course!" we said, laughing.) The fact that we were completely unprepared for the weather conditions and we ended up uncomfortable and soaking wet as a result. ("My shoes and socks are so wet that I can hear them squishing," she said with a grin.) The fact that my friend didn't have pockets, so she ended up putting her phone into the waistband of her pants, where it eventually slid down to a much less desirable place at one point. (To which we howled with laughter and were grateful that she didn't end up taking a picture with it.)

I've said it many times before: It's all in how you look at it. It didn't occur to either one of us to be angry or upset about the situation. But I know plenty of people who would have taken this unfortunate turn of events to get perturbed, ticked off, annoyed, or self-pitying, and they would have made sure that everyone they talked to over the next week knew about the rotten thing that happened. Some people I know would have used it as an excuse to complain about how the bad things always happen to them, to focus on how unlucky they are, and to quote Murphy's Law as their own perpetual creed.

Personally, I don't have time for any of that. Was I cold and wet for about thirty minutes of my life? Yes. Are my shoes going to take a good two days to dry out? Probably. Was it how I had planned for this part of my day to go? Nope. But so what? Yes, I got caught unexpectedly in a rainstorm complete with hail, but I got to laugh about it with a dear friend and it's one of those unpredicted and hilariously funny experiences that becomes a happy memory to look back on with a smile.

We can apply "So what?" to so many experiences that don't go the way we wanted or that are surprisingly unpleasant. The unexpected traffic jam, the extra-long line at the DMV, the inclement weather when we had planned a special outdoor event—no one enjoys these things, especially because they remind us how out of our personal control these things are in our lives. In these times, we absolutely have the choice to laugh at it and make the best of it, or to get upset by it and have it potentially ruin our entire day. This isn't easy to do when pessimism is our default setting, but stopping in the middle of what has gone wrong, taking note that it's not as bad as it seems, and then choosing to say something to ourselves like, "So what?" or "It really doesn't matter so much" can cause a shift in our very existence. It can turn a frustrating situation into something that's manageable and bearable, and depending on what's happening, you can even turn it into something funny and laughable. It becomes you taking control of the situation in the best possible way you can.

So, the next time something unexpectedly unfortunate happens to you, make the choice to find the humor in it, or at least to *not* find the misery in it. Make the choice to laugh in the rain, no matter what happens to your shoes, or where your phone ends up.

Comparison Is the Death of Joy

That's a quote from Mark Twain and it is the truth. We are taught from a very young age what is "better" about other people and how they compare to us. There are the "cool" kids in school, and the "lucky ones" whom everyone else wants to emulate. There are the "hot" toys and gadgets and clothes of the season that everyone has to have, or we are "less than" by comparison. We compare ourselves with others in our looks, the amount in our paychecks, the size and location of our homes, and in what we do with our time every day. I would venture to say that most of the time when we compare ourselves to others, we come up short, no matter how happy we actually are or how confident we feel in the choices we have made for ourselves. What a jaded and miserable way to live.

Here's the really interesting thing about comparing yourself to other people and what is deemed "acceptable" or "desirable" by the current society: **The standards of greatness and beauty and power and accomplishment CHANGE.** It's like moving the goalposts. There is a standard that people choose to measure themselves by according to the time and place they're living in, but those standards can vary drastically, which is something that we all need to remember when we start playing the comparison game.

I recently saw Bo Derek speak about her age and her looks. (If you who don't know who she is, in the late 1970s and early 1980s she was considered to be one of the most beautiful women on the planet with the ideal body that all women should strive to have.) She was well aware of the effect her presence had on women in those days but was also very cognizant of her luck at becoming so famous and worshipped for her looks. She said, "I realize that I have the right body type and the right bones for now; a couple hundred years ago I would have been the scullery maid—the scrawny, skinny girl." Isn't that fascinating? She would have been undesirable back then because the standard of attractiveness was based on a woman's perceived ability to bear children, which would have meant having a curvier figure.

Here's something that also occurred to me recently: For the past few decades what has been presented through us in the media is that if you're successful then you're rich, and if you're rich then you own a big house (or several) and you fill up those big houses with stuff. The more stuff you have, the better and more successful you are. Well, now there is a whole minimalist and tiny house craze and people with a lot of material things are being judged negatively for having too much. On the one hand, everyone wishes they were celebrities with their palatial homes, but at the same time, people are being shamed for trying to emulate that level of wealth and accumulation.

I won't even get into different beauty and status standards in other countries, or how they can vary from state to state, town to town, and even from street to street. It's really absurd how everyone judges everyone else because of what they were taught to believe at some point or what they were brought up to believe that "society" deems best on a superficial level.

We can't ever truly be happy if we fall into the comparison trap. So how do we break free? By focusing our energy and attention on what we are doing ourselves to live the happiest life we can. By reminding ourselves that what someone else is doing with their life has nothing to do with fulfilling our own goals and potential. No one is born inherently better than anyone else, and no one becomes better because they meet some predetermined artificial standards set by advertising executives and the media.

The best way to not compare ourselves to others is to be so captivated by our own lives that we don't have the time or inclination to look at or wish for anyone else's.

It is possible to live happily in the
here and now. So many conditions of
happiness are available—more than
enough for you to be happy right now.
You don't have to run into the future
in order to get more.

—THICH NHAT HANH

Patience Is a Choice

Patience is not the ability to wait
but how you act while you're waiting.
—Joyce Meyer

I just had to share my experience from today. It was a huge lesson in choosing happiness, joy, and patience instead of frustration, anger, and irritation.

I arrived at my alternate post office this morning (I was doing errands in the next town over) about ten minutes before it opened. I was fourth in line and it was a rather jovial bunch in the small vestibule, as we chatted amiably about how early we all were and the impending snow coming later in the week, just in time for Mother's Day. (I know, I live in a crazy place.)

When the door finally opened at a few minutes after nine, there was but one lowly postal worker behind the counter. She started taking people one at a time, and through no fault of her own, she was as slow as, as they say, molasses in January. (Or for me, here in Colorado, apparently molasses in mid-May.) She was just one of those people who moves in slow motion, no matter what she's doing. Five minutes go by, ten minutes go by, and then the person in front of me goes up, and she's mailing a package to Poland.

Now not only does Bernadette behind the counter have to deal with the overseas customs form, she also has to type in the recipient's name and address, which is not an easy task because they are long and unfamiliar. She kept typing them into the computer incorrectly and the woman mailing the package kept correcting her, and then they began having a lengthy conversation about what was inside the package ("Oh, it's a dress? What kind of dress? For a girl or a woman? And a sweater too? What kind of sweater is it?") At this point the customer politely asked Bernadette, "How come there is only one of you working today? There is quite a long line."

By this time there was indeed a very long line of customers waiting. There were about ten people behind me, most of whom were getting very fed up with the lack of effective customer service exhibited here.

There was sighing, there were repeated checks of wristwatches, there was significant shifting of weight from one foot to the other. These were accompanied by major eye rolls, more audible sighing, and knowing glances and head shakes exchanged with one another as if to say, "Can you believe the utter incompetence that we have to deal with?"

About the time that the foreign street name was being spelled out for the third time I felt myself begin to get one of the most intense hot flashes I have ever had. I felt the burning start in my neck and come up to my face, and pretty soon rivers of sweat started pouring down my face. I took off my outer jacket, then my sweater, then began fanning my t-shirt-clad self with one of my smaller packages. At that point the whole situation just seemed so absurd to me and I started giggling to myself. My giggling turned into laughing, and considering my entire face was probably beet red I'm certain that my fellow line mates thought I was having some kind of episode.

Anyway, eventually someone else finally came out to the counter to help (the lovely Polish woman was still at the counter, now describing the gift of the shoes) and I went up, slightly cooler by now, but still amused by the whole turn of events that had transpired since I'd arrived.

Let me rephrase that: **I made the choice to be amused by the whole turn of events that had transpired since I'd arrived.**

I could have gotten upset and angry and frustrated at how incredibly slowly the line was moving and how truly "trying-hard-but-it-just-wasn't-her-day" inept Bernadette was. But I made the conscious choice to remind myself that I was not particularly in a hurry, that I would be taken care of eventually, that standing in a crowded post office fanning myself wildly was still a better place to be in than a lot of other places, and nothing was going wrong. I was just a little inconvenienced, as were all of the people behind me who were choosing ire over joy.

I'm not saying I'm so great here, I'm just pointing out that in almost every difficult situation, if we can't control what's happening, we can at least control our attitude while we're going through it.

When it comes to patience, I believe that for those of us for whom it does not come naturally, it is a skill that can be practiced and learned. It's about calming down, keeping your mind in the present, realizing and acknowledging the hopefully non-severity of the situation, and most importantly, doing our best to see the humor in it. Getting angry and frustrated certainly doesn't make a line move any faster, it just makes us that much more grumpy, and who wants that in their life?

Practice patience when you can and when it's necessary. And when you have to, find a different post office.

Keep Things in Perspective

What's the opposite of a superpower? Would that be a curse? Well, today I was reminded of the curse that I have had since I was a young child—the curse of never getting a good haircut.

That's not exactly true. I have had exactly two haircuts that I have been completely happy with, which were done by a stylist in a different state from where I lived, hence it has only happened twice. Usually I'm pretty satisfied with what the stylist has done, but oftentimes when they have finished and I look into the mirror, it's a disaster.

I am aware that this is most definitely a first world problem, but like they say in season two, episode five, of *Fleabag*, "Hair is EVERYTHING! I know it shouldn't be, BUT IT IS!"

Suffice it to say that I have had my share of hair disasters—the wrong color, cutting it way too short, leaving it too long, and my most recent experience of telling the stylist that I was growing my bangs out, only to have him snip off the three months of painstaking growth as I was reminding him not to do so.

Again, I know that in the grand scheme of things this is really nothing to be upset about, but after this particular experience I just felt frustrated and angry that nine times out of ten when I sit in a stylist's chair I ended up feeling disrespected, with my requests completely ignored.

I grumbled my way to the car in full "why does this always happen to me?" self-pity mode and headed to the post office. (Yes, I go there a lot.)

I got in line, still kind of muttering to myself about the injustices of the world and my hair's place in it, when I glanced up at the woman in front of me. She was sporting a haircut that was white and about half an inch long. She also walked with a limp and had pale ashy skin, so while it's possible that her hairstyle was by her own choice, I made an educated guess that it wasn't.

In that instant I remembered the family friend who was diagnosed with breast cancer last week and was talking to my relative about wigs because she was about to lose all of her hair due to upcoming chemo treatments. I also thought about the many women I have known who have not only lost their hair but their lives to a similar diagnosis, and I felt tears start to brim in my eyes at the thought of them, as well as the thought of how utterly ridiculous I was acting.

Thank You, Universe, for that much-needed perspective exactly when I needed it.

Hair is important. But a bad hair day, or a bad hair few weeks, is never something to get super upset about. **Hair grows.** No matter how bad it looks, it instantly starts growing again—so it is never, ever permanent.

We can apply this to things besides our hair too. Did we make an embarrassing mistake at work? Luckily time marches on and it will be forgotten soon enough. Did we spend money that we shouldn't have, on something we regret? Hopefully we will keep going to work and make enough money to cover the expense, and it will be a good reminder to not make that same mistake again. Did we say the wrong thing to someone and need to apologize? Luckily there is always a new day in which we can forge a new path, go through a different door, and make amends to help us start afresh.

It's so important to keep a healthy perspective about things in life. It's all in how we choose to look at them. Even when things make us angry or disappointed or frustrated or sad, we can still make the choice to rise above them and not let them ruin our day.

We have the power over what is going to affect us in our daily lives. Take hold of that power, and choose happiness, no matter what our hair looks like, no matter what our bodies look like, no matter what we have to do, who has disappointed us, or what chapter of life we might be in on a given day.

In the meantime, do you have a good hair stylist you can recommend?

Choosing Happiness Means Choosing Tolerance and Acceptance over Racism and Prejudice

Seriously.

The other day when I cut my finger in the kitchen, I had an epiphany. Thankfully it was a small cut and I immediately did what my physician friend had told me years ago—cover it, apply tight pressure, hold it above your heart, and don't look at it for five minutes straight. (Thank you, Dr. Rob.)

As I stood there for that time, my mind went to the marvel-inducing fact that every single person on the entire planet bleeds when their skin is cut by a sharp object. And the blood that they bleed is red.

So that got me thinking about other similarities that all human beings have. Like:

When a person's heart stops beating, they die.

Every. Single. Human. Being.

When dust flies up a person's nose they involuntarily sneeze.

Every. Single. Human. Being.

With rare exception, when a person loses someone they love, they feel grief.

And the biggie—every single human being who has ever lived, who lives now, and most likely will ever live, was created in the same way.

Every. Single. Human. Being.

This is one of the reasons why I will never understand racism. Or bigotry. Or prejudice against any other human being. It doesn't make sense to me, because we are all so much more similar than we are different. We may think differently, we may love differently, we may feel things differently, but on the most basic level, every single human being's bodily functions are the same. I would add that on an emotional level, every single human being wants to live without fear, without discrimination, without neglect, and without indifference. I would argue that just about every human being to some degree wants to feel joy, to feel love, to feel seen, and to be free to live the live that she or he wants to live.

If fundamentally we're more alike than we are different, then why do people hate each other that they've never met and that they don't even know?

I honestly couldn't tell you. What I can tell you is that people whose lives are filled with hatred for their fellow human beings have no room for true happiness. They were probably taught their beliefs in childhood, which might make those opinions as ingrained in them as breathing. But to me, this is no excuse. There is enough information out in the world to dispel the myths that one kind of person is superior to another, and if in today's age a person still chooses to be prejudiced then that is squarely on them; I don't care how they were raised.

Ultimately the only person I can control is myself, which is why I am determined to speak up whenever I see racism or discrimination perpetrated in my presence. Part of my happiness depends on me doing the right thing for my fellow human beings, who bleed the same color as I do and who understand what it feels like to be victimized and mistreated.

Which brings me to ...

There Is Only One Race, the Human Race

"The lesson I want you to learn is: It doesn't matter what you look like. You can be tall or short or fat or thin, or ugly or handsome, like your father, or you can be black or yellow or white. It doesn't matter. But what does matter is the size of your heart and the strength of your character."*

These are lines spoken by Herman Munster, played by Fred Gwynne on an episode of *The Munsters* that aired on January 28, 1965. The video clip has been going around the Internet as people are struggling with the latest and all-too familiar incidents of blatant racism and prejudice taking place on the streets of the United States. And even though the quote above uses old descriptive words that are inherently prejudicial, they are not used to be pejorative, which is an important distinction to be made. The message of the quote is clear—**it doesn't matter what you look like, what matters is the person you are on the inside.**

People like to say that the issues of racism are complicated, but I don't believe that. I believe that no matter how you look at it, racism and prejudice against any other human being are wrong and always will be. There was never, is never, and never

---

*Writing credits from *The Munsters*, season 1, episode 19, "Eddie's Nickname." Written by Richard Baer, developed by Norm Liebmann and Ed Haas, from a format by Allan Burns and Chris Hayward.

will be any reason for one human being to denounce another human being.

Why?

Because no matter what point racist people will try to make to explain their views, the following things are true for every human being on the planet:

When a human being gets cut anywhere on the body, it bleeds. And the blood is red. (I know I said that before, but it bears repeating.)

Every human being (with rare exception) has a heart that pumps that blood to vital organs including one liver, one pancreas, two lungs, one stomach, and one brain. **Every human being.**

Every human being breathes in oxygen and breathes out carbon dioxide.

Every human being needs that oxygen to stay alive.

Every human being was born from two parents.

Every human being was a baby once, who couldn't walk or talk or feed itself.

Every human being has to eat food to stay alive.

Every human being has to process waste and eliminate it from the body.

Every human being (save anomaly cases) shares the same brain chemicals that trigger laughter at something considered funny and cause feelings of emotional pain when experiencing grief.

Every human being, no matter how they speak, how they were raised, where they work, how they choose to spend their free time, what they believe in, or what they look like, deserves respect, decency, and compassion.

Because here is something else that's a fact: Every single human being who currently has the precious gift of life will have that gift taken away one day and will die. Make no mistake, that's **every human being.**

Simply knowing that fact and recognizing it should help us all to realize that no matter how our lives began or how they are going, we all meet the same end. So why would anyone spend even one second of that time alive putting a fellow human being down or treating them any other way than we'd like to be treated ourselves?

No matter what a person was taught or what was propagated to a person at some point, the following statements are true:

Racism is a choice.

Prejudice is a choice.

Discrimination is a choice.

Sexism is a choice.

Xenophobia is a choice.

But these are also true:

Love is a choice.

Compassion is a choice.

Kindness is a choice.

Tolerance is a choice.

Empathy is a choice.

And yes, happiness is most definitely a choice.

What will your choice be?

Embrace What Makes You, You

> *Cherish what makes you unique*
> *'cuz you're really a yawn if it goes.*
> —Bette Midler

In a book by Mr. Rogers, he talks about witnessing a cello class taught by the amazing Yo-Yo Ma. After one of the students had finished playing a piece, Yo-Yo said to him, "No one else can make the sound that you make." That applied to everyone in the class and to every single one of us as well. No one else has our unique talents and gifts to share with the world, and only each of us has our own distinctive story to tell in our own individual voice. Which I think is something to be celebrated!

So why do so many of us strive to be "just like everyone else?" As if there is a standard somewhere out there that would make us acceptable or worthy because we fit perfectly into it. This is why hair gets dyed, freckles get bleached, and Spanx are uncomfortably squeezed into. It is also why spouses, jobs, and locations are often chosen not because they fulfill something necessary within us, but because they are the "right" ones, deemed by our idea of what that "rightness" is. (Usually determined by someone else's opinion.)

Throughout my life people have felt the overwhelming need to tell me my flaws directly to my face. I have been told I'm too loud, too boisterous, too generous, too nice, too fat, too noisy, too much fun, too considerate, too clumsy, too quick, too sweet, too organized, too encouraging, too hard working, too dramatic, and too caring.

(Let me address the "too nice/too considerate" epithet for a second here. Is there some "nice and considerate" meter out there that says that a certain amount is acceptable, but then there is a point where someone can go over that quantity and the scale tips over into the objectionable range? What is the algorithm for that and what factors does it take into account?)

I have also been told on many occasions that I am "not enough" of certain desirable things. Not thin enough, not pretty enough, not athletic enough, not talented enough, not bitchy enough, not sedate enough, not tall enough, not tidy enough, not organized enough, and not quiet enough.

It seems that no matter how I live my life, some people are always going to find fault with me.

Which is the point here. None of us fit perfectly into whatever magic mold is out there that people seem to think is ideal. We are ALL unique, and designed to be different from each other, because that is what makes life interesting and how things get done in the world. There's a reason why we all shudder at those scenes in the post-apocalyptic movies where all of the people look exactly expressionlessly alike, wearing the same prison-issue clothes, trudging slowly along a dimly lit hallway in perfectly straight lines, intoning the same chant with lifeless eyes and immobile arms.

And yet this concept of homogeneity is what social media and magazines and red carpets constantly tell us we need to conform to. We allow models and movie stars, many of whom lead lonely and personally unfulfilled lives, to dictate what we should love about ourselves, and what we desperately need to change.

A big part of choosing happiness is choosing to love the skin we're in and embracing what makes us stand out from the crowd. We have to choose to see our uniqueness as the miraculous gift that is and concentrate on what only we can say uniquely in our own voice. There is only one you, there is only one me, and there will never be the exact combination of those genes and traits repeated ever again. How cool is that?

So never be ashamed of yourself or about anything having to do with what you look like or how you are. Choose to celebrate and revel in the fact that you are exactly how you are supposed to be and that you are utterly and wholly magnificent in your own way and in every way.

Just a Very Few Thoughts on Money

People say that money is not the key to happiness,
but I always figured, if you have enough money,
you can have a key made.
—Joan Rivers

I would never, ever give another person advice on how to spend their money. Money is a very personal thing, and people have very different ideas about spending money and saving money and making money and losing money and everything in between. Of course, I can only offer opinions based on my experience, and what I've observed in my years of living so far. So, all I will share are the few things that I've learned that I believe are valuable when it comes to money and its relationship to our happiness.

1. Avoid getting into debt, especially credit card debt. I knew a woman who owed more than $30,000 on credit cards because of her obsession with designer shoes and purses. Her debt became crippling and invasive into every aspect of her life including her marriage and her ability to be a stable parent. I knew another woman who started her own business by putting everything on her credit cards and only paying the minimum balance every month. Within two years she had

to declare bankruptcy, which carries with it a nearly lifelong sentence of denials for things like purchasing a home or having a healthy credit score. Money can really cause long-lasting problems for us if we don't use it wisely.

2. To that end I would say to spend your money on experiences and other people, rather than just on things. As I stated in the chapter "Keep Household Clutter under Control," while some things can definitely bring us joy, no material possession can ever provide the very basic human need of being seen, validated, acknowledged, and loved. This is something important to keep in mind when we get an unexpected windfall or late-night online shopping beckons.

3. Save early, save often. Start putting money away for your retirement as early as you can and always have an emergency fund that you can draw upon if necessary. There are thousands of books and articles on this subject, but I just thought I'd mention it here because while saving money may seem difficult and depriving, making the choice to do it can make a big difference between long-term strife and long-term happiness, especially in our golden years.

4. Don't save all of your money at the expense of happiness either though. I know a lot of obsessively frugal people, who will forgo necessities they can easily afford, like a window air conditioning unit to provide relief during a dangerously hot and humid summer, because by their calculations it costs too much money to purchase and to run. By doing this, these people put their health and happiness in jeopardy by putting the monetary price above their daily well-being. Yes, saving money is important and essential, but it should never take precedence over health, safety, or common sense.

I also knew someone who longed to travel. He yearned to see faraway lands and experience other cultures firsthand. His parents lived through the Great Depression and taught him that saving money was tantamount, and that none should be spent except for the absolute essentials in life. When this man passed away he had a lot of money in the bank, but took his greatest dreams with him in death. As a wonderfully wise woman I knew, Dona Hochart, used to say, "You'll never see a safe following a hearse."

Money can be a very effective tool for helping us accomplish our goals and making our dreams come true. It can also be a heavy burden to bear when we don't use it as a helpful instrument toward those things. We all need to assess the choices we make around spending money and reassess them periodically as our needs and options change throughout our lives. You don't need to follow the same rules that your parents exhibited—as a grown-up you can take what you were taught and adapt those lessons into what works for you and your life choices now.

Lastly, just a quick reminder that "you can't take it with you," as they say. Money should be shared, in whatever capacity is possible, with those that need it. Giving money away to others—through gifts, charitable monetary or in-kind donations, and other contributions can bring us enormous amounts of joy throughout our lives when we are able to do it. One of my favorite movie lines ever comes from the classic musical *Hello Dolly!*: "Money, pardon the expression, is like manure. It's not worth a thing unless it's spread around encouraging young things to grow."

When we're choosing happiness, we need to remember to save our money wisely, spend our money wisely, and share our money wisely. It absolutely cannot buy happiness—and it behooves us to always remember that our self-worth has nothing to do with our net worth.

The Best Revenge
Is No Revenge

As I have said before, many people in my life have been mean to me. Work colleagues, hard-hearted people masquerading as friends, even some family members. I have had countless people feel the overwhelming need to tell me what I'm doing is wrong, how my choices are incorrect, and at times, how horrible I've looked. It no longer surprises me how people who claim to be well-meaning will say insulting and demeaning things directly to a person's face—specifically MY face—that I would never even dream of saying to another human being, much less think them in the first place.

Over the years I have learned that these people's acidic remarks have nothing to do with me; rather, it has to do with their own misery and unrelenting feelings of unhappiness. Putting someone else down, especially someone who chooses to look at the world with optimism and hope, somehow makes them feel better about themselves and their perpetually bleak outlook on life. While I know this to be true, sometimes that realization doesn't fully take the sting out of a comment or a judgment made by someone whom I have chosen to trust and who purports to have my best interests at heart.

Many years ago, I saw something that said, "The best revenge is a happy life." I like that concept, because it goes along with the old "sticks and stones" or "I'm rubber and you're glue" schoolyard sayings in response to a bully's taunts. If we can ignore the bad things that people say to us to try to bring us down to their sad and hopeless level, then we will rise above their meanness and not give them the satisfaction of making us more like them. In short, we get back at them, by doing the opposite of what they want.

But now I have a different way of looking at this. How about if we remove the part about "getting back at them" in the first place? Instead of taking in what these people say to us and turning it around, what if we didn't even allow it to enter our consciousness at all? What if we didn't give the bullies and the naysayers and the discouragers even one ounce of our attention or acknowledgment? How about instead of saying, "How dare they say that to me, I'll show 'em!" and giving them even one iota of power over our own decisions and our own lives, we simply dismiss them as not the people that we need right now in our circle of support and move on immediately? That shifts the power from them and their vitriol, to us and our strength and unfailing belief in ourselves and our own abundant sense of worth.

When we assign someone else too much authority over our lives, then whatever they say, good or bad, can have far too much of an impact over what we know in our hearts and minds to be true. If someone compliments us on an outfit we're wearing, or a haircut, or on something we've artistically created, those things can automatically get vaulted into the category of something that we like more or something that we're more proud of, regardless of how we actually feel about it. Then the outfit becomes "The One That People Said I Look Good In," instead of "The One That I Like and That Makes

Me Feel Good In." See the difference? By the same token, I've had clothes that I've loved that people have made rude comments to me about (horizontal stripes, anyone?) and as a result they have been relegated to the back of my closet or given away immediately, because now they have this other person's negative opinion attached to it. Why on earth should I care what someone else says about something I own that I love? Why should I attach any amount of importance to what they think and what they, for some unknown reason, need to tell me about it?

The point is, the concept of revenge continues to put the power into the hands of the offending person. When people spend their time daydreaming about how to exact revenge on the person who has wronged them, they are using up precious time and energy on someone who does not deserve even a millisecond more of their mental and physical bandwidth. Planning revenge against someone gives that person exactly what they wanted in the first place: to bring you down to their level of anger, disappointment, frustration, contempt, and misery. Resentment, vengeance, vindictiveness, and spite are all choices that we make ourselves, and while they might seem comforting in the moment, they are not a recipe for a happy and fulfilling life.

So while I used to think that the best revenge against someone who has wronged me was to live my happiest life possible, I now believe that the best revenge is no revenge, which keeps my power where it belongs; in my own heart, in my own mind, and firmly rooted in my own happiness.

We cannot cure the world of sorrows

but we can choose to live in joy.

—JOSEPH CAMPBELL

Just a Few Thoughts on Anger

Choosing happiness means letting go of anger. There's no Venn diagram that shows happiness and anger overlapping (well, unless you're a sociopath, I guess).

I am a firm believer that as Ralph Waldo Emerson said, *For every minute you remain angry you give up sixty seconds of peace of mind.*

However, in recent times, my mind has changed a bit on that, and I have found that sometimes there are benefits from a healthy anger. Healthy anger to me means that we are so fed up and frustrated by the injustices and blatant inequality in the world that we cannot wait one more moment to do something tangible about it. In those cases, our anger can be fuel for getting important things done that are vital to the survival of others.

The Civil Rights Movement, Women's suffrage, Black Lives Matter, #Metoo, and #Timesup are great examples of people's anger being turned into action. But it's important to remember that while anger can be the catalyst for revolution, it has no place in the actual demonstration of the need for systemic change. We don't need one more life lost or one more precious human being injured in the name of what should be basic human decency and fairness.

While usually anger can be poison to our soul, peaceful action from righteous anger can be the antidote. Choosing happiness for ourselves needs to mean that everyone, and I mean EVERYONE, has the chance to choose happiness for themselves as well.

Never Give Up Your Power

Ever.

Yesterday was a tough day for my feelings. I had two phone conversations and one email exchange in which all three of the people I was dealing with insulted me, said rude things, and were inconsiderate and demeaning overall. Both phone calls took place right after each other, and by the time I hung up with the second I was not in a good place.

I was hurt, angry, disappointed, annoyed, and most of all, frustrated that these people—who claim to love me and have my best interests at heart—felt the tremendous need to disrespect me for the umpteenth time. I remained upset about all of these encounters and kept wondering if there was any way to handle them that wouldn't escalate matters and make them worse.

After about an hour, I had a revelation that hit me completely out of the blue but is one that I will carry with me for the rest of my life.

Why am I continuing to give power to people whose opinions and views I do not respect?

Moreover, why am I continuing to give power to people who clearly do not respect me or my opinions?

Constructive criticism is one thing. When people care about you and want what's best for you, sometimes it's their job to let you know if you're going off the rails in certain aspects of your life. That's what friends are for at times, and hopefully those gentle suggestions are presented from the perspective of wanting you to be as happy and fulfilled as possible in your life.

I'm not talking about that. I'm talking about the people who can only see life through their own critical lenses and who feel the overwhelming need to correct other people's behaviors if they do not line up with their own. These people are not coming from a place of caring about YOU, they are coming from their own place of insecurity and an immense need for their own viewpoints to be heard.

When these people spew their thoughts and opinions over everyone who will give them the time to do so, we have two choices:

1. We can choose to take what they say to heart and allow their put-downs and condescension to ruin our days and our happiness.

OR:

2. We can choose to ignore what they say, and look at them as the sad, miserable, always-trying-to-prove-themselves-even-though-no-one-asked people that they are, and not let their words or actions affect us one bit. We don't need to be rude back; instead we can listen respectfully, treat them the way we'd like to be treated, and then move on with our heads held high, persevering in our power instead of relinquishing it to those who don't deserve even the tiniest bit of it.

This goes back to the whole "sticks and stones" thing, but I want to make it clear that **you and I have permission** to disregard what someone says to us, even if they are close friends or family members. This is more than just name calling on a playground. When we are choosing happiness in our lives, we are wholly allowed to make the choice of whose advice we listen to, whose opinions we seek out, and who we ultimately let into our hearts, minds, and souls.

We each have the power to decide how we're going to live our lives, and that power is YOURS. Own it, stand in it, revel in it, and wield it when you have to, to preserve your own happiness—no matter who or what might be trying to take it away from you.

Take Your Power Back, and Keep It

The past has no power over the present moment.
—Eckhart Tolle

In my work with abuse victims I have noticed one thing that most of them seem to share. They are carrying their abuse around with them like another limb, and they continue to let the abuse define themselves and the decisions they make in their lives. Even if the abuse happened decades ago and the perpetrators no longer share the Earth with their prey. One man in particular had just turned fifty, and he placed the blame for him not having any successful relationships, for his several failed businesses, and for his lack of close friends squarely on his alcoholic and abusive father, who had been deceased for more than ten years by this point. He was no longer being terrorized by anyone, but he was still letting the horrible things that happened to him long ago completely rule over his life.

I knew a woman who at age sixty-eight still talked about her long-dead parents and the abuse she suffered at the hands of both of them as if it was still going on. Whenever she brought up her childhood, her eyes filled with tears and she experienced the cruelty over and over again as if she was still the frightened five-year-old going through it. She believed that it was impossible to get over what happened to her, and likewise blamed her upbringing for the many disappointments in her life.

While I honestly understand this behavior—I do, I get it—I also believe that no matter what happened to us as children, we as adults get to choose what we focus on in the years after the abuse ends. We can choose to rise above our circumstances and no longer suffer for things that should not be causing us pain.

How can we do this? Here's one exercise that I have found to be helpful.

When a memory of abuse comes up, stop what you are doing and ask yourself these questions:

Was what happened to me horrible?

Answer: Yes!

Was what happened to me wrong?

Answer: Yes! Absolutely!

Was what happened to me unfair, unjust, and unwarranted?

Answer: Yes! One hundred percent all of those things.

Do I have the right to be upset about what happened to me?

Answer: Yes, as much as I want and need to be.

Is it true that what happened to me was not my fault?

Answer: Yes! A thousand times yes!

It's important to validate our feelings and our right to feel them at this moment in time.

Then ask yourself these questions:

Does what happened to me then have to affect my life as it is now?

Answer: No. No it does not. Not one iota.

Does what happened to me have to have anything to do with the decisions I make as an adult?

Answer: No. No it does not.

Does what happened to me have to define me and my actions for even one moment more?

Answer: No. No it does not, even for one moment more.

It is equally important to invalidate the abuser and the abuser's power over your life for this moment in time.

It is vitally important to note that when we allow our torments from the past to negatively affect our present and our future, **we are now doing it to ourselves.** The abuser is no longer doing it to us, we have taken up their emotional weapons and continued their attempts to hurt us of our own volition. In short, we are still giving that person or people immense power over our lives, which we do not need to do! As adults we have permission to make our own choices and leave the old and destructive behaviors far in the past where they belong.

It is utterly heartbreaking that when the abuse comes from a parent or a close trusted family member, the victims often hold on to their abuse tightly because they still seek the love and approval from that family member that they had yearned for. By continuing to live out the abuse and the consequences of it, they are honoring the abuser's memory by still reacting in the victimized way that was expected of them. In doing this they believe that they are somehow going to finally get the unconditional affection and love they have always needed. Consciously breaking free from that childhood longing is essential to building a truly happy life, which means no longer needing those voids to be filled by ghosts from the past.

Here's another exercise that can be helpful:

I know a woman who at age forty-five told me that she was sexually abused three times during her teens. She was subsequently unable to have any kind of meaningful emotional or sexual relationship with a partner, which was devastating to her, since her deepest desires were to be married and have children. The three incidents, which were horrible and overwhelmingly damaging emotionally, kept her from making her dreams come true.

Please understand I am not discounting the magnitude of these instances in any way, but in order to recover from them, perhaps they can be viewed in a detached, scientific way.

The average time of each encounter was approximately five minutes.

If we multiply three incidents times five minutes that's fifteen minutes.

At the age of forty-five, this woman had been on the Earth for, give or take, twenty-three million, six hundred and fifty-two thousand minutes. If you take away the fifteen minutes of the abuse, then you could say that there were twenty-three million, six hundred and fifty-one thousand, nine hundred and eighty-five minutes that she had lived so far when she was NOT being abused. She was allowing those fifteen minutes—those terrible and horrifying fifteen minutes—to take over the more than twenty-three million, six hundred and fifty-one thousand minutes she had also lived. It's kind of staggering when you look at it that way.

This kind of exercise isn't for everyone, but it could be a way of evaluating thoughts that take up tremendous amounts of mental energy and that can have long-lasting destructive consequences. Seeing the relativity of time can possibly open a door to freedom from the things in our past that hold us back from living the happiest and healthiest lives we deserve.

The simple truth is, no matter what has happened to us in our past, we have the choice, starting at this very moment, to become the person that we have always wanted to be. We can decide what thoughts take up our daily bandwidth, and we can choose true happiness for ourselves, regardless of how many times we were told to choose otherwise.

> *The only person you are destined to be*
> *is the person you decide to become.*
> —Ralph Waldo Emerson

We Do Not Have to Succumb to Sadness

We really don't. I know some people who wear their misery like a badge of honor. They believe that the more upset, angry, and stressed out they are, they more they are living "real life," and all of the terrible things that come with it. They take a lot of pride in being a martyr, and they enjoy telling others about their suffering in great and significant detail.

I have to say, I have no time for these people. It seems like they are trying to show the world that they care more about the state of things because they are choosing to be so indignant about everything all the time. They cannot understand how anyone can find the good in anything because they themselves cannot seem to find anything but bad, bad, bad everywhere they look.

In a way it's easier to just look at the bad stuff and resign yourself to things never getting any better. It takes strength to foster things like hope and joy and optimism in our lives, especially when the daily news is telling us otherwise.

It all comes down to mindset. Yes, terrible things happen. Yes, we get disappointed and crushed and beaten down. Yes, there is a lot to be sad and upset about at any given moment. But if we want to choose a different path for ourselves, one of joy and light and gratitude, then I would encourage you to think about this:

I don't think of all the misery,
but of the beauty that still remains.
—Anne Frank

Here's the funny thing about seeing the bad side of every-thing: **It doesn't make anything better.** The people who wallow in sadness and despair believe that by acting this way, they are somehow improving the situation. They also tend to believe that it makes them superior, and if other people aren't reacting with the same negative attitude then those other people are wrong.

Being around these outwardly negative and critical people is endlessly tiring.

I'm not saying that we shouldn't be affected by things—we're not sociopaths. In difficult times we need to give ourselves ample space and time to experience sadness, grief, and pain. They are all a part of living, and learning how to deal with hard things is how we can ultimately move on from them. But therein lies the key: we have to MOVE ON. We do not have to let the bad feelings overtake and consume our daily lives forever. It doesn't do any good, no matter what the people who cling to them might tell us.

Pain is certain, suffering is optional.
—Buddha

Make the choice to acknowledge your pain but keep your suffering to a minimum. We all have the ability to make that choice, and it's absolutely essential to experiencing a healthy and happy life rather than a miserable one.

Which do you prefer?

Being Alone Does Not Have to Mean Loneliness

I just wanted to remind you if you're going through a lonesome patch that **being alone does not have to equal being lonely.**

For a born extrovert like myself, I get happy energy and recharge my batteries from being with other people. The very act of being social gets my proverbial juices flowing and revs me up with adrenaline and inspiration. For dyed-in-the-wool introverts like my husband, you all find refreshment and renewal in being away from people, and if you don't get enough solitude it can be as bad for your health as sleep deprivation.

Neither one of these is wrong, it's just a different way of being, biologically. And I believe that while we have been designed a certain way from birth, it is possible to change one's extrovert/introvert leopard's spots with practice and time. My husband has learned over the years how to be extroverted and social when necessary, and I have found that I am able to happily embrace my solitude and even appreciate it as something good when I feel bombarded by outside stimuli.

I'm writing this during the COVID-19 pandemic quarantine, where people around the world have been isolated for many months without contact with friends and family members. Lots of us have been craving human interaction and necessary comforting touch from hugs and handshakes. It's a bizarre time, when we can't even see smiles on people's masked faces nor connect in any social ways other than from a safe distance outside.

So, what can we do to combat the loneliness and despair from such limited human contact? **We can make it happen for ourselves whenever and however we can.** We can reconnect with people with whom we have regrettably lost touch through phone calls, video chats, and online meetings. We can make the effort to write handwritten letters to loved ones, and we can even go old school and make new "Pen Pal" friends. I can remember running excitedly to the mailbox during my childhood to see if there was a letter there from my Pen Pal across the country. There is nothing like having something fun and uplifting like that to look forward to, and to know that someone else is thinking of us from somewhere far away.

In our world right now, we have neighbors who have been dropping off flowers from their garden on everyone's porches once a month. It's a tiny thing, but believe me, it makes a big difference in the humdrum of life right now. We ourselves have been making regular porch deliveries of gifts and baked goods to people whom we know are isolated from their families and friends. Don't underestimate the power of reaching out to someone else when they are lonely; doing so will bring you right out of your own loneliness like a rainbow after a storm.

Being alone can be lonely, no question about it. And so many studies have shown how loneliness can be crippling and devastating to our minds and bodies. Human beings are social creatures by nature, and having to be cut off from our biological requirement of socialization can have debilitating effects. So, make the choice to not allow yourself to drown in the dark ocean of loneliness. Kick your way up to the surface, take a deep breath of fresh air and keep swimming your way toward others on the friendly shore.

It may be uncomfortable at first to reach out to others but remember that we are all in the same boat here, we're all human beings trying to make the best lives we can for ourselves in the short time we're here on Earth. We're honestly all in this together and no one needs to be lonely even while being alone. Make the choice, take the step, and reach out to connect with fellow kindred spirits on our shared journey toward happiness.

Have Fun!

Never underestimate the importance of having fun.
—Randy Pausch

Having fun is one of the most important things we can do in our lives. People might think it's frivolous, people might think it's childish, people might think it's immature, and people might think that it's something that sophisticated, educated, and classy people don't do.

Well, let me ask you this question: Has anyone ever looked back on their life and bemoaned, "If only I'd had LESS fun?"

Kids know how to have fun instinctually, and then we lose that predisposition as we age, either because people reprimand us for not acting properly or because somewhere along the line we picked up the training that fun was something to be had only on certain occasions and the rest of the time we were to take things as seriously as possible once we hit a certain age.

Because having fun makes us happy, it seems like oftentimes we crave things like whimsy and entertainment to bump up the fun meter in our lives. This is why if you take a look around places like Disney World and amusements parks there are often far more adults attending than children. This is why we go to concerts and parties and celebrate holidays—because we want and need to have FUN!

In my opinion, fun isn't something to be scoffed at for any reason. I've mentioned before when people have said to me when laughing in public, "You're just having way too much fun." Again, I ask, "Is that possible?"

I remember seeing one of my idols, Julia Child, on a talk show. She was re-creating her very first television appearance by making an omelet on a hot plate in the middle of the studio. Instead of using a spatula to fold the eggs over, she began shaking the pan vigorously toward herself, and away from herself, and toward herself again. The host asked her, "Why do it this way?" Julia replied gleefully,

"Because it's fun!"

Always remember that doing something "just for fun" is a perfectly valid reason for doing it. Ignore the people who think that fun is overrated or reserved just for children. These people seem to embrace the opposite of fun, which according to the dictionary is misery and boredom. Who wants to live like that?

Life is what you make it, so make it fun and the happiness will follow in abundance.

Forgiveness Is Key

> *To forgive is to set a prisoner free and*
> *discover that prisoner was you.*
> —Lewis B. Smedes

Forgiveness can be a tricky thing. For the longest time I thought that forgiving a person and/or their actions meant that I was giving them absolution for what they did and therefore saying that what they did was acceptable.

Then over the years I kept coming across quotes like this:

Forgiveness doesn't mean that what someone did was okay . . . it means that YOU'RE okay.

And:

Resentment is like drinking poison and expecting the other person to die.

And:

Holding on to anger is like grasping a hot coal with the intent of throwing it at someone else; you are the one who gets burned.

Those pithy statements make it sound like letting go of resentment and anger toward someone who has hurt us is a simple thing that any of us can do as easily as flipping a switch. Like, Anger: OFF, Forgiveness: ON. Well I can tell you that as much as we might like that to happen, that's not how it works.

But I can also tell you that true forgiveness is freedom. It opens the door to happiness, and if that is what we're choosing

in our lives, then **we have to make the choice** to let go of resentment and bitterness toward others.

This concept crystallized with me the other day when a
friend of mine texted me to ask if I had a minute to talk. This
was unusual in our relationship, so I called her immediately,
fearing something was wrong. She launched into a lengthy
apology, saying how sorry she was for offending me and how
she didn't mean for what she said to come out like it did and
she went on and on and ended with "Can you ever forgive
me?"

It was such a heartfelt and lovely apology, which I really
appreciated (since I know how difficult it can be to apologize
to someone), but part of me was really confused because **I had
absolutely no idea what she was talking about.**

Seriously. She was explaining in detail about how she had
been feeling guilty for weeks about something she had said in
an offhand way at a get-together and it hadn't even registered
as offensive to me in any way.

She was super relieved, and we moved on with our conversation, and after we hung up, I spent the next few hours
thinking about the whole thing. The following things came
to mind.

1. It struck me that there had been many other times that
   this friend had actually offended me to my face, but
   those never seemed to bother her. I didn't understand
   why this off-the-cuff (and thoughtless, now that she
   mentioned it) statement made her feel so badly.

2. She had been carrying these bad feelings of guilt around
   with her for weeks and it wasn't even on my radar. To
   flip it around, how often do we ourselves carry around

things that we have perceived someone did to us deliberately, when the hurt they may have caused was not intentional and they had no idea that what they said or did was harmful?

3. Whether or not we get offended by something is our own choice. It's the whole "Teflon" thing. Just because someone says or does something mean or disrespectful **does not mean that we have to take it that way.** The fact is, we can have the inner power and resilience to NOT let that person's rudeness or utter lack of consideration ruffle our feathers in any way.

Another important thing to note here is that forgiving is by no means forgetting. There are plenty of people whom I have forgiven, but I have also taken steps to make sure that there are minimal chances for them to do something to me that I would then have to forgive them for again. The unfortunate occurrences that happen between people can be great life lessons for us in dealing with them, and the sooner we learn how to let things go that get in the way of our happiness, the better.

It takes strength to be able to forgive something or someone and to move on healthily and happily. I find that it's the weak people who hold grudges and replay personal offenses over and over in their minds, sometimes for years on end, hoping that somehow those practices will lead to some kind of resolution or satisfaction. I can tell you unequivocally, they never do.

Most folks are about as happy as

they make up their minds to be.

—ABRAHAM LINCOLN

Don't Get Bitter . . . Get Better

When you harbor bitterness, happiness will dock elsewhere.
—Andy Rooney

This is hard. No one's saying it's easy. But in order to choose happiness, we need to rally against those things that, according to the dictionary definition of bitter, make us "angry, hurt, or resentful because of one's bad experiences or a sense of unjust treatment."

So how do we do this? I personally can say that I have been more disappointed, hurt, and angry as a result of other people's actions more than I have been satisfied or contented with them, especially when I have needed something important. As a result, you would think that I would have become inured to this, and honestly, I wish I could tell you that I am. But there's a part of me that still wants to see the best in other people and trust that when someone says they will help me they will actually come through with what they promised. As much as I would like to squelch that impulse of hope within me sometimes, I do not want live my life as a perpetually miserable person always expecting the worst. As much as an optimistic attitude might disappoint me in the end, I still think it's a better way to be.

Here are some things I have learned from dealing with these potentially bitterness-inducing situations:

1. Do not take mistreatment personally. That is very difficult to do, because the hard truth is, people put their time and effort into things that are priorities for them. When they don't follow through with what they say they are going to do, it clearly shows that something else has taken precedence over what you need. That can really hurt, especially when you have done your part to be a good friend or relative to this person, even going out of your way to help them when they needed it. Been. There. More times than I can count. But you have to remember that their choice to not reciprocate has less to do with you than it does to do with them. While I personally can never understand how someone can feel perfectly fine going back on a promise, many people have no problem doing that at all, which shows us something important about the nature of their character and provides an opportunity for us to question whether or not we really want this person in our lives. Sometimes it's good to get the proverbial "kick in the head" that we need to help us see a person's value (or non-value) as it pertains to our happiness and well-being.

2. When you're done being justifiably angry and frustrated and upset, pick your head up and move on. DO NOT LET THIS PERSON CLOUD YOUR JOY OR DULL YOUR SHINE FOR ONE MORE MINUTE OF YOUR LIFE! This is really important because we can get stuck in "I can't believe they took

advantage of me again!" or "How come nobody is ever there for me when I need them?" or "Why is it always ME who has to go out of my way when no one else reciprocates?" These feelings are all real and warranted, and you have full permission to feel them. So feel them and **then let them go** so you can go on with your life as happily and freely as possible. Instead of simmering in the resentment, get out of yourself and focus on better things.

3. Something that always helps me out of bitterness is getting outside. Physically breathing in fresh air, looking up at the sky, and getting myself immersed in nature reminds me that there is a bigger world out there outside of my disappointments.

4. It also may help to make a list of all of the people in your life that you CAN count on, instead of focusing all of your energies on those you can't. Even if the list is short, it's a good reminder that this one disappointing person is not the entire be all and end all of your world; you DO have people who support you and love you and consistently put you on their priority list.

5. Another thing that you can do, which may seem petty and unnecessary (but what I have found to actually be cathartic and healing), is to get rid of material things that remind you of the person causing your bitterness. I'm not saying to put everything out on your lawn and light it on fire a la Angela Bassett in *Waiting to Exhale* (although I do love that scene), but when you do something tangible that represents finally getting this person out of your life, it can be very freeing. I knew someone who suffered a devastating spousal betrayal

and after a few months of grieving she realized the situation for what it was, without so much emotional baggage attached to it. At that point she was ready to take some kind of palpable action to help her get over the unrelenting and immobilizing pain. So she gathered up all of the gifts and letters she had received from her husband and threw them away, relishing watching the garbage truck come and remove them from her life forever. These kinds of actions are just that—ACTIONS—that we can take, to reassert our power over our lives and to consciously and deliberately reaffirm ourselves of our own strength, worth, and authority.

Bitterness can be a safe and comfortable hole to hide in while we're nursing hurt feelings. But please don't stay down in there for too long. You have too much good to offer this world, to let someone else's words or actions control how you're going to spend your day. I cannot impress upon you enough how important it is to fight the bitterness and make another choice as often as you can. Choose freedom, choose joy, and choose peace, which can only be found in light instead of in darkness.

In the beautiful words of Nelson Mandela:

> *As I walked out the door toward the gate that would lead to my freedom, I knew if I didn't leave my bitterness and hatred behind, I'd still be in prison.*

Amen.

Music Is Magic

Have you ever seen people at a concert, singing all of the words to a song at the same time? Maybe with their hands up in the air, swaying back and forth all together? It can be a truly spiritual experience.

Why?

Because as Sir Paul McCartney put it: *That's the power of music.*

Music can evoke emotions in us on a visceral and primal level, much like a certain smell or taste will instantly transport us back in time to when those sensory experiences represented something important for us.

Have you ever been moved to tears because of a song? Has a song ever made you want to stand up and cheer? Does hearing a particular song make you feel closer to a friend or family member? Do certain songs make you feel inspired or strong or unstoppable?

Athletes often use music to pump themselves up before a race or tournament or big game. The image of Olympic swimmer Michael Phelps and his headphones comes to mind. Ancient warriors would sing songs and beat tattoos on drums to help get them ready for battle. And there's a reason why babies fall asleep so easily to lullabies. Indeed, music contains powerful magic inside of it.

So, if you don't have a magic wand handy, I would suggest that you turn to music when you need help in choosing happiness for yourself. Figure out your "battle songs" for when you need confidence to put yourself out there to try something new. Learn what your "salve songs" are, for when you need to calm down and escape from the pressures that life is throwing at you. Keep as many songs as you want handy for different situations that you're dealing with, and feel free to change them up as you're introduced to new songs that evoke significant feelings within you.

Even more fun is to have your own "theme song." I saw this concept years ago on the TV show *Ally McBeal*. Tracey Ullman played Ally's therapist and suggested that Ally adopt a theme song for herself when she needed to be reminded of her own power and worth. She suggested that Ally listen to it or play it in her head during upsetting or stressful situations to help turn herself around and feel better. She assured Ally of the benefits of this practice, and that she herself had utilized a theme song since she was ten, announcing emphatically "it still works!"

I'm here to tell you, IT DOES! I have my own theme song, and every time I hear it, I'm re-energized, I'm encouraged, and my spirits are instantly lifted, no matter what else has been going on. It's kind of amazing, actually.

Shakespeare famously said, *If music be the food of love, play on.*

Hans Christian Andersen said, *Where words fail, music speaks.*

Henry Wadsworth Longfellow said, *Music is the language of mankind.*

Henry David Thoreau said, *When I hear music, I fear no danger. I am invulnerable. I see no foe. I am related to the earliest times, and to the latest.*

And to quote Dumbledore, *Ah music,* he said, wiping his eyes, *A magic beyond all we do here.*

I could go on and on about the transformative power of music, but I will close here with this:

> *Music will help dissolve your perplexities and purify your character and sensibilities, and in time of care and sorrow, will keep a fountain of joy alive in you.*
> —Dietrich Bonhoeffer

Keep that fountain of joy alive in you whenever you can. Choose your music to help you choose happiness.

Stop Stewing
in Your Own Juices

There are a lot of ways to say this: Get out of your own head. Get out of your own way. If you don't like something, change it. I particularly like the image of us marinating in a giant pot of our own misery because I think it's a powerful one that can hopefully cause a positive change in our behavior.

What exactly do I mean by this? I mean, don't get so caught up in focusing on what you're unhappy about, and letting that get you so down that you're unable to do anything about it. For some of us, it's replaying injustices done to us in the past. For some of us it's desperately wanting to make a change but not feeling confident enough to step out of our comfort zone. For some of us it's knowing what we're doing is making us unhappy but it's such a comfortable old habit that we lack the emotional resources and wherewithal to break it. And for some of us, we'd just rather "stew" in our own suffering.

Here's an example: I knew a woman who had just turned forty. (She is now in her late fifties and spoiler alert, nothing has changed.) She would bemoan the fact that she was still single, she would complain about how she could never meet anybody, and she would go on and on about how upset and frustrated she was by this. What was she doing to help the situation? Was she going to meet-and-greets for singles on the weekends? Was she joining activity clubs to increase the chances that she'd meet someone with similar interests? Did she regularly ask friends and family to set her up with single people they knew? Nope, nope, and nope. She was doing none of these things, and with her inaction she was *choosing to remain miserable*. In fact, on some level I think she must have enjoyed being unhappy because she never once took even one step to mitigate it.

That's stewing in your own juices.

Another example: I know a lot of people who worry constantly, as if the act of worrying is something active rather than passive. They turn things over and over in their heads, perseverating constantly over what could go wrong, what might go wrong, and what will inevitably definitely go wrong, all the while never trying to come up with a solution to what they are worrying about it. Most of these people end up with serious health problems as a result of such profound anxiety, and they live their lives in a state of incessant fretting borne of their own thoughts.

They're stewing in their own juices.

Here's my point: **If you want to choose happiness then you have to un-choose unhappiness.** Make the choice every day to stop the tape in your head and to take the steps toward the happy life you truly want. Get out of your stew and throw away the pot for good. The juices in there are old and gross and are really really bad for you.

Emotional Scar Gel

A few years ago, my daughter fell and had to get stitches in her knee. She now has a sizable scar just below her right kneecap. As the gash was healing, we got her scar gel, a topical application which is supposed to "reduce the appearance, color, and texture of scars." I am so glad that there is a product out there that can diminish the effects of physical scars. But what do we do about mental and spiritual scars, which run much deeper and cause more long-lasting pain?

Emotional scar gel is harder to find because it has to come from within us instead of on a shelf at the drugstore. It CAN be found within our hearts and our minds however, in the form of things like:

Forgiveness.

Joy.

Laughter.

Hugs.

Hope.

Belief in a better tomorrow.

Opening up yourself to receiving love.

Doing what makes you happy.

Following a passion.

Having faith in something bigger than yourself.

Putting the past behind you once and for all.

Yes, you have every right to be upset, angry, frustrated, indignant, sad, and vengeful about how you were treated and what happened to you. It was cruel, wrong, unjust, unfair, painful, undeserved, and unjustified. But feeling those feelings every day instead of feeling happy and hopeful about the life you have created for yourself now only leaves you flailing around in all of that sadness and despair that was caused a long time ago. Or even a short time ago. By clinging to those scars and what caused them, you have no freedom to pursue love or creativity or true happiness. You are essentially living in the scar, instead of in the healing tissue growing around it.

Look at professional surfer Bethany Hamilton. She lost her entire left arm to a shark attack. Did she let herself be defined by that immense and incredibly conspicuous physical scar? Not even a little bit. She returned to surfing one month after the attack, kept training and winning surfing competitions, plus she wrote a bestselling book, has appeared on multiple television shows, had a major motion picture made about her life, and played herself in an inspirational documentary film. Along with all of that, she also fell in love, got married, and gave birth to a son in 2015.

If she had given up surfing, given up competing, given up on her once planned-out life, it would have been an expected and reasonable reaction to what happened to her. In short, she got a free pass to let her disfigurement define her and her future. My guess is she would have been unhappy and unfulfilled every day, letting the scar rule her life and make all of her decisions for her, regardless of what her mind and heart desired.

She is the perfect example of someone who moved past her injury to immense success and chosen joy. Each of us has sustained injuries, especially emotional ones, and if we are able to move past them by administering our own emotional scar gel, then we don't have to allow outside circumstances to determine our ultimate happiness or well-being.

Scarring is a natural part of the healing process. And scars can be a good reminder to not put ourselves into harm's way. But every scar is proof that we *can survive* whatever life throws at us, and that we are able to truly heal and move on from each one.

What Do You Want on Your Tombstone?

I guess that's kind of a grim way to put it. Maybe a better question is, "What do you want your legacy to be?"

Of course, none of us really knows what our actual legacy will be because that is up to other people and how they remember us. But if it's important to us to leave some kind of legacy behind, it is vital that we take the steps in our lives to hopefully create the legacy that we want. Very few of us will have big, physical things left behind like buildings with our names on them or awards created in our names, so what are those other, more intangible things we'd like people to remember us by? In other words, how would we like our proverbial tombstones to read (since in reality, we're not getting much more than our name, date of birth, date of death, and a little dash in-between those two about an inch long)?

What are we taught in our society about what makes a successful life, defined as a "good" life, or a "life well lived?" What are we told are the things to aspire to that will signify our worth in the world? Three things come to mind: To be rich, to be famous, and to be beautiful/good looking, which in our country equals slender, muscular, toned, and symmetrical.

Let's unpack those for a moment, shall we?

There is an inherent assumption that we've had a good life if we were rich. The more houses, cars, and fancy vacations we've accumulated has a direct ratio to how successful we must be. And while it is true that all of these things can definitely make us happy on some level, I would argue that these trappings of wealth almost always come at a price.

In my pre-kids career as an events planner I met some very rich people. We're talking extreme wealth, with multiple homes, each with its own full staff for both the house and the grounds. In all of these cases, the men worked ceaselessly outside the home, while the wives took care of the children and pursued their own volunteer projects, sitting on arts council boards and things like that. Interestingly, in the three families that I worked most closely with, they each had four kids, and all three of the husbands ended up trading in their wives for younger models after about twenty years of marriage. While I don't know anything else about these exceedingly affluent men, it seems that their main accomplishment in life was their material wealth, so each of their imaginary tombstones would read "I Was Rich." Maybe some people would love that as their epitaph, but how important is that as a legacy really, do you think?

Let's look at being famous. Some years ago, I had an encounter with someone who had achieved a considerable amount of fame in his youth. He talked about how he was so well-known at one point that when he was walking around a mall, he had to buy a baseball hat and sunglasses because people kept accosting him for autographs and photos every few steps.

"Wow!" I said, "That must have been great!"

He looked at me for a moment and replied, "It's not as great as you think."

He went on to explain how lonely his life was back then, because he couldn't go out in public much, and didn't have many real friends because all of the people he knew were phony, show business–type people. He admitted that the money was nice, but he was too young to really know what to do with it, and as a result of some bad financial decisions, that money was gone and he was having trouble finding work due to the difficulty of making the transition from child star to adult actor. At this point he was divorced, had limited visitation with his kids, and looked back on his years of fame with regret and some bitterness.

This reminds me of the line from the film *Notting Hill* where the ultra-famous character played by Julia Roberts bemoans what she see as her upcoming future, *And, one day not long from now, my looks will go, they will discover I can't act and I will become some sad middle-aged woman who looks a bit like someone who was famous for a while.*

For all of the people who yearn for millions of "likes" on their social media videos and who want nothing more than to be famous, it's important to remember that fame is entirely dependent on *what other people think of you.* Is that really something to base a whole life on? Does "I Was Famous" make a satisfying tombstone inscription?

And now to the topic that takes up immense amounts of our mental and physical bandwidth: What we look like and how it compares to what is considered the standard for socially acceptable beauty at this point in time. I have a former friend I used to call "Pageant Patti." (Complete with a little star dotting the "i.") She was a Southern woman who participated in pageants in her youth and when you arrived at her house, before you even took your coat off she would direct you to the glass case that held all of her tiaras and sashes, which was in front of the wall covered with her pageant photos. They were all from more than two decades ago, but I got the impression that every morning when she came down the stairs she would stop and gaze at that shrine, reliving her glory days from long ago.

Even in her forties she still looked like a Barbie doll. Naturally petite, long wavy blond hair, perfect teeth, and a body that literally looks good in everything she wears. We became friends for a few years while our kids were on the same sports team, and as we would talk, I realized how often the conversation became focused on her obsession with her looks, her body, and what she was doing to determinedly outwit Mother Nature and Father Time.

I heard about the Botox injections to combat the crow's feet from years of tanning beds for the perfect pageant tan. She talked at length about her week-long liquid diet before a company holiday party, where her then husband chose her outfit and instructed her on how to purposefully mingle with the higher-ups who would be there. She was always trying new workout regimens and posting "before and after" bikini photos online, craving as many "thumbs ups" and approving comments as possible. She also had regular salon appointments for highlights, hair extensions, manicures, and pedicures, plus body waxings, exfoliations, and polishes.

From her enviable looks alone, one would assume that she had the perfect life. I must admit that when I first met I her I was jealous of her ideal appearance and the opportunities I presumed she had gotten as a result it. As it turns out, the burden of constantly trying to preserve her youthful beauty had a cost to other aspects of her life.

She had been divorced twice (first husband was a serial cheater, second one was an emotional abuser), she was estranged from her family, and at one point was in so much debt she was on the verge of becoming homeless. She had nearly no close friends and was not a person whom you would call warm or considerate. All of her energy was put toward maintaining her "pageant perfect" looks, and her entire life's focus was her obsession about it. If we added up all of the hours spent devoted to that endeavor, her tombstone would definitely read, "I Was Pretty."

I loved hearing an interview with actress and director Tracee Ellis Ross, who made a point of saying that she does not answer questions about her diet or her workout regimen because, she said, raising her voice, *"THERE ARE SO MANY MORE IMPORTANT THINGS TO TALK ABOUT THAN WHAT I LOOK LIKE!"*

It has been said that if you want to see what a person really cares about, just look at his or her daily activities, bank statements, and the people around them. We spend our time, money, and effort on the things that matter to us, regardless of what we may claim otherwise.

So I ask you, what do you want your epitaph to be? How would you like to be remembered? Is it time to question the qualities and factors that society and social media deem "successful?" What does a "good life lived" mean to you? Maybe try looking inside at what fills you up based on what you inherently love and not what someone else tells you is "correct" and what you "should" aspire to. It turns out that being rich, famous, and pretty are not the magic answers to a happy life, and the sooner we figure that out, the happier our lives will be.

Turn your grumbles into gratitude.

Trade your expectation for appreciation.

Thankfulness is happiness.

—RACHEL COLE

A Counter Thought to Choosing Happiness

In my interview with Dr. Brian Emerson,* founder and CEO of the leadership coaching company Riverstone Endeavors, he brought up something that really gave me pause, especially with regard to my intention of encouraging others to consciously choose happiness.

What do we do when no matter how hard we try, we *cannot* choose happiness?

There are times in our lives when we are submerged under an avalanche of grief, or when we are in nearly unbearable physical or emotional pain, when the concept of happiness feels like it is completely out of reach, and impossible to ever feel again. During those times, what can we choose instead? What is an option that will leave us feeling even a tiny bit better, or micro-incrementally stronger, or the teeniest morsel uplifted when we most need it?

His advice? Choose gratitude. His example was, if he was in an insurmountable state of grief (i.e., losing a parent) he was pretty sure that he would not be able to choose happiness during that time. But he believed that something helpful he *could* choose was to be grateful. Grateful for the time he had with that parent, grateful for the memories of times they

*Brian's company can be found at www.riverstoneendeavors.com.

shared together, and grateful for the relationship they'd had over so many years.

This is really a fantastic concept because the truth is, there are going to be some days, or some stretches of time, when life throws something at us that is unbelievably difficult to deal with, and in those times, happiness can be elusive or disappear altogether.

I can remember a time when I felt like I was drowning in grief and despair, so much so that I was doubtful that I'd ever feel true happiness again. What did I choose then?

I chose contentment. I couldn't be happy, but I could be content with what I was left with after the loss I experienced. For me, contentment means realizing and recognizing what I have—very similar to gratitude—and accepting it as enough. Yes, I lost someone very close to me, but what kept me afloat was focusing on what I *hadn't* lost, what still remained, and labeling it as sufficient for me to be content and okay.

In those devastating times, maybe something else we can choose is peace. We can try our best to stay calm and center ourselves by taking deep breaths and consciously feeling our feet grounded to the floor. We may not be able to conjure up any feelings of joy, but we can hopefully take steps to get ourselves to a state of serenity in the midst of a difficult situation.

Choosing happiness isn't easy, nor is it simple. Even when everything is going well for us in our lives, it's still so much easier sometimes to focus on the bad and remain in our comfortable cocoon of misery. It takes work to choose happiness sometimes, but it's work that is meaningful, that can change our lives for the better, and is therefore worthy of our time and effort.

The Dalai Lama said, *The purpose of our lives is to be happy.* I couldn't agree more. If we start with that intention, then everything will fall into place behind that beacon. We just need to keep our eyes on it as much as possible to have the happiest and most fulfilling lives that we can, even when it seems like we can't.

An Innovative Way to
Start the Day

This concept also comes courtesy of Dr. Brian Emerson.

We have all heard about how important gratitude is in creating and keeping a happy life. We've heard about gratitude journals, and saying our "Gratefuls" out loud, beginning our day with what we're grateful for and ending our day with thankfulness. I am a big believer in all of these things, and I encourage you to make gratitude a daily practice because it can truly be a life changer and a lifesaver.

In accordance with making these a part of our daily morning and evening routines, I would also encourage you to add in things that you are looking forward to, especially in the morning as you start a new day. As I have said before, having something to look forward to can make the difference between having a truly happy life and one of mere existence. So, if we put together the concepts of gratitude and joyful anticipation, what if we started every day by asking ourselves this question:

What am I looking forward to being grateful for today?

This is different from just asking "What I am looking forward to?" because it sets the intention that we're going to have something so wonderful happen today that it will make our list of "Gratefuls" at the end of the day. It also puts us in the mindset of making sure to do or experience that thing and notice it happening. This keeps us in the present moment

beautifully and helps us to acknowledge the happily anticipated thing as it's taking place.

Brilliant.

It's a good day to have a good day. And a great day to have
something to be grateful for.

When Life Hands You an Opportunity, Take It!

My family and I were touring the ancient ruins of Pompeii and when we got to the amphitheater, our tour guide showed us the ancient "sound check" by standing in the exact middle and clapping her hands. You could hear the sound bounce off of the walls and reverberate all around—it was super cool. Then she looked at me and said, "Try it, sing something." (She did not know I was a singer.) I was like, "What? Here? Now?" She said, "Yeah, sing!" I replied, "I don't know any Italian songs." To which she shrugged and said, "Sing anyway."

In that moment, time stopped for a second, and then everything went into slow motion. I stepped into the center of the floor, looked around at the magnificent architecture from thousands of years ago, and realized in an instant that this opportunity was never going to come again. I took a deep breath, opened my mouth, and did what I was born to do.

It was astounding. My voice soared and took flight over the stones and into the sky. Tour guides stopped speaking. It grew quiet around me and some people took out their phones and started recording. It was one of those magical moments suspended in time and space, and I'll tell you, those ancient Romans knew what they were doing when it came to acoustics.

I sang the first two verses of "Somewhere over the Rainbow." I chose something that I thought most people would know and that had a simple melody. When I was finished everyone applauded, I took a little bow, and then my family and I moved on to the next place to see. As we left, a man leaned over to me and whispered, "Thank you for giving us that opportunity."

Opportunity indeed.

Now I am not sharing this to say how great and talented I am. I just wanted to share that when the Universe presents you with an amazing opportunity, TAKE IT! I didn't think about how awful and sweaty I looked in the moment, I didn't stop to check my hair before I started singing, I didn't worry about a key or if I would be able to hit the notes, I just DID IT, and it became a tiny piece of history that a bunch of complete strangers got to share together, far away from our regular lives.

I don't have a video of it, it happened so fast, but here is a photo of the moment when life presented me with a brass ring, and I grabbed it for all I was worth.

To quote Fausto, a very kind Italian man we met, *"Life is short! We believe in enjoying it as much as we can!"*

Si si si! Life is short indeed. When it gives you a chance, take it!

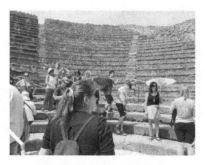

Me in Pompeii, June 2019

Don't Give Up

Don't give up, there'll be plenty of time to give up later.
—Jake Johannsen

It's easy to give up, isn't it? It's comfortable, it's simple, and it's usually effortless. But it's also disappointing, discouraging, unexciting, boring, and doesn't ever get us to our goals.

It can be easy to lose hope during difficult times, and it's in those times that we have to reach out for it, grab it, and hold onto it as tightly as we can.

There are so many things that we try that are impossible to master the first time. Swimming, riding a bike, ice skating, walking on a tightrope, long-distance running, to name a few. Even things that don't take particular physical skill or coordination like cooking, computer coding, and playing a musical instrument all require patience, repetition, and sustained learning over a long period of time, combined with the desire to succeed that supersedes the often overwhelming wish to give up.

This applies to mentally and spiritually giving up as well. Sometimes we get stuck in a rut of seeing things pessimistically and thinking that hope is a waste of time and mental effort. In those times we have to practice being hopeful, the same way we would practice an instrument or a new language in order to get to some measure of mastery.

How can we do this? By consciously reforming the thoughts in our minds from negative ones to positive ones. By making the conscious choice to take the steps we need to pull ourselves out of the dark pit we've gotten ourselves buried into. By viewing the world as a place of light and possibility, no matter what the news headlines say.

Like happiness, hope is a choice. We always have the opportunity to choose hope over despair and optimism over pessimism.

We really do.

I hope you always will.

Additional References for Choosing Happiness

BOOKS

Joyful: The Surprising Power of Ordinary Things to Create Extraordinary Happiness, by Ingrid Fetell Lee

The Blue Zones of Happiness: Lessons from the World's Happiest People, by Dan Buettner

Gift from the Sea, by Anne Morrow Lindbergh

The Art of Possibility, by Benjamin and Rosamund Zander

Improvisation for the Spirit: Live a More Creative, Spontaneous, and Courageous Life Using the Tools of Improv Comedy, by Katie Goodman

Let Your Life Speak, by Parker J. Palmer

When Things Fall Apart, by Pema Chodron

I Wish You More, by Amy Krouse Rosenthal

14,000 Things to Be Happy About, by Barbara Ann Kipfer

Simple Abundance: 365 Days to a Balanced and Joyful Life, by Sarah Ban Breathnach

TV/ONLINE SHOWS TO GENERATE LAUGHTER

Impractical Jokers, https://www.trutv.com/shows/impractical-jokers

RiffTrax, www.rifftrax.com

The Marx Brothers, https://www.marx-brothers.org

The Carol Burnett Show, especially the blooper reels, https://
    www.shoutfactorytv.com/series/the-carxol-burnett-show
The Muppets, https://muppets.disney.com/
Jake Johannsen, www.jakethis.com
Comedians in Cars Getting Coffee, www.netflix.com
Victor Borge, www.victorborge.org

PODCASTS
The Happiness Lab, www.happinesslab.fm
Wait, Wait, Don't Tell Me, https://www.npr.org/podcasts/
    344098539/wait-wait-don-t-tell-me

Acknowledgments

Thank you to Jane Raese, book designer extraordinaire. I could not have done this without you, and I am tremendously grateful for all of your help and guidance in making this book a reality.

A huge thank you to all of the subscribers to my Choose Happiness videos and blogs. You have been there with me since the beginning, and I so appreciate your support and encouragement along the way.

Thank you to my interviewees to date: Dr. Brian Emerson at Riverstone Endeavors, www.riverstoneendeavorscom, Robert Kramer at www.kramerleadership.com, Kristin Massotto, Edson Jeune at CoachWithEdson@Yahoo.com, Shy Ashkenazi at www.facebook.com/Shy-Ashkenazi, Parrish Salyers at www.pscreativeco.com, and Carlo Sciortino at http://voyagela.com/interview/meet-carlo-sciortino-hollywood. I continue to learn from your advice and insights, and I am forever grateful for your time and for sharing your ideas and viewpoints so magnificently.

Interviews can be found on Youtube: www.youtube.com/channel/UC8bzWp99WXRLhhm3kwTNffQ.

Or search Rachel Cole Choose Happiness.

And at www.choose-happiness.net.

Thank you to Dom Testa for your inspiration and your encouragement. Your writing career and your emboldening words during a live writing presentation at the Denver Public Library were the catalyst for this book. www.domtesta.com

Thank you to Jake Johannsen for all of the laughs, life-long quotes, your immense talent, and your considerate heart. I appreciate you and all that you do to bring happiness to the world. www.jakethis.com

Thank you to the illustrious, joy-inducing Kristin Massotto for being such a pure source of happiness for me for so many years.

Thank you to Rob Kramer for all of your advice and counsel through the years, and for the healing power of shared laughter that you always provide.

Thank you to Liz Christensen for always being there to listen on a walk (even in the pouring rain) and for being such a fantastic cheerleader to me in all of my endeavors.

Thank you to Michelle Welsh-Horst for your superlative friendship, your ever-appreciated and unending encouragement and support, as well as your stellar book publishing advice and knowledge.

Thank you to Ben for always bringing the joy with you wherever you go and for reminding me of what true happiness looks like.

Thank you to Sarah for all of your help with this project and for providing me with immeasurable opportunities for choosing laughter and joy (even at the DMV) in my life.

Thank you to Jason for always believing in me, inspiring me, lifting me up, and for showing me how to see and choose hope, possibility, and happiness every day.

www.choose-happiness.net

About the Author

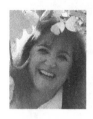

Rachel Cole is an award-winning singer/ songwriter, recording artist and performer. Additional professional endeavors have included teacher, events planner, workshop leader, librarian, and for a short time in high school, retail sales associate. Along with spearheading the Choose Happiness project, Rachel owns and runs a gift-giving business and is the founder of a nonprofit organization that provides wedding dresses and formalwear to women and girls in need. Rachel also wears the titles of mom (her #1 favorite job), wife, sister, daughter, aunt, niece, and friend, all of which she takes very seriously and honorifically.

The Choose Happiness project came about when Rachel became an empty nester and her daily mom duties were majorly reduced. She was looking for a way to fulfill her lifelong goal of making a positive difference in the world around her, and through a series of events (including a chance encounter at the post office) the idea of providing weekly videos and blogs to promote the concept that happiness is a choice was born. The content is based on experiences from her own life, combined with interviews from people from around the world who make happiness a priority in their lives. Rachel believes very strongly that we can all make the choice to see the good over the bad, to choose hope over despair, and to seek peace in spite of pain. Life is short and it's up to us to choose happiness purposefully and intentionally, and to do so as often as we can.

www.choose-happiness.net